No One Ever Told Me . . .

A collection of motherhood stories to get you through your *postpartum* journey.

No One Ever Told Me . . . : A Collection of Motherhood Stories to Get You Through Your Postpartum Journey

YGTMedia Co. Press Trade Paperback Edition

Published in Canada, for Global Distribution by YGTMedia Co.

www.ygtmedia.co/publishing

ISBN paperback: 978-1-998754-00-7

To order additional copies of this book: publishing@ygtmedia.co

Developmentally edited by David Lipson

Book design by Doris Chung

Cover design by Michelle Fairbanks

Printed in North America

No One Ever Told Me . . .

A collection of motherhood stories to get you through your *postpartum* journey.

Jordana *Handler* & Lani *Lipson*

We would like to acknowledge the people who helped birth and nurture this project.

To our partners who supported us and held down the fort while we brought this vision to life. David Lipson and Jonny Handler, we are grateful for you.

To our babies who taught us to share our own stories and set this train in motion, Noa, Ophelia, Delilah, and Judah.

To our community of mamas who shared stories, support and love with us over the last few years, we acknowledge your vulnerability and honesty in creating a conversation that all new moms can be a part of.

And to Greer who introduced us back in 2014 and changed our motherhood experience forever.

NO ONE EVER TOLD ME…

INTRODUCTION

Changing the *postpartum* conversation,
one story at a time

Sleep deprivation, depression, "poonamis," psychotic in-laws, loneliness, leaky breasts, and bad sex. Welcome to the fourth trimester, a.k.a. 100 days of hell. During this period following childbirth, there is so much wonderful care and attention directed to newborns, but we moms often get left behind. Motherhood is a new reality that many of us are unprepared for because we lack the vital information needed to face the physical, mental, and emotional challenges it brings. There are so many things that no one ever tells you about being a new mom. Four years ago, we set out to change that by giving women an opportunity to share their truths about motherhood—the real stuff that often gets glossed over on social media. Consider this book the essential survival guide for navigating the fourth trimester—something to make the first 100 days a little less hellish.

Our hope is that reading these stories will remind you that YOU ARE NOT ALONE. Whether you relate to one story or all of them, it's so important for you all to know that even when it feels the loneliest or as if you're the only one out there going through your experience, there are so many other new mamas in your situation feeling the same feelings. We want to validate your feelings, no matter what stage of postpartum you're in. When we give mothers permission to be honest and honor their bodies and feelings, we open the door for positive postpartum experiences. The first step is conversations that don't tiptoe around the real struggles and triumphs of being a mother.

Not Just for Moms

Just as a new mom can read these stories and feel less alone, their partner or family members can read them and learn how to be more empathetic and supportive. A new baby puts an enormous amount of stress on relationships. We heard numerous accounts of moms "hating" their partners, friends, parents, and in-laws. We're not claiming this book is a panacea for family friction, but it will definitely help.

How to Read the Book

The stories we collected fall into many categories, but we tried to divide up the content as much as possible into sections that have a similar theme. As you go through the stories, you will be invited to share your own experiences through prompts. It might feel strange at first, but we HIGHLY encourage you to write your story through the prompts. You will be amazed by how putting words to your experience can help you process and move through your postpartum journey in new ways. There are, of course, some heavier sections that touch on topics like miscarriage, loss, mental health, or the physical/mental health of the baby. We will always note them with a trigger warning, and we welcome you to skip them if you don't feel ready or willing to read them.

Online Support

If you don't already follow us on social, you can find us on @this.is.eemah on Instagram. Through our platform, we connect, share, laugh (sometimes cry), and mostly support each other through a growing community of moms (and sometimes dads) who want the honest, no bullshit truth about the fourth trimester and postpartum experience. We also go further beyond the first four months after giving birth because the struggles and triumphs that new moms face go beyond those four months. Come follow along to connect with moms in your shoes and ones who have done a bit of the walk already. Wherever you are in your journey, you are welcome.

Thank you,

Jord & Lani

1

NO ONE EVER TOLD ME
ABOUT RECOVERY. PERIOD.

Everyone around you is wearing white pants one
week out, and you're still in diapers? We see you.

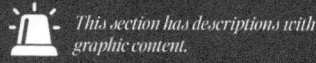 *This section has descriptions with
graphic content.*

*N**o one ever tells you how fucking uncomfortable you're going to be in an adult diaper.*** I had a C-section, and I was so sore. Getting up and moving anywhere was hard. There were a few times when I couldn't make it to the bathroom. I fully peed in my pants and the bed. It was not okay. You don't even notice when you're in the hospital because they give you those massive pillow-sized pads, but then you come home and a regular pad isn't doing it.

I had to take the baby to the pediatrician within the first few days, and I stopped on the way home to buy adult diapers. There are so many to choose from. I was standing there in the adult diaper aisle comparing the brands and what they do. This one is ultra-absorbent, but this one lasts for nine hours, and I was thinking . . . what the fuck have I done with my life? There is just no shame at that point. I had to suck it up and wear a diaper. My husband and I laughed about it, but he also fully saw his wife in an adult diaper, waddling around the house and peeing in her pants. I'm really glad we're married and he is stuck with me now, because that was not an attractive sight.

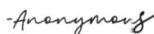
-Anonymous

My delivery wasn't straightforward. My labor was fine, but when I was ready to push, my baby's heart rate dropped. I saw the room filling up with doctors, all trying to figure out what to do, and within fifteen minutes, they tried both vacuuming and forceps and ended up doing an episiotomy and putting the forceps back in. I watched the whole thing, and I have no idea how they fit those things up there. It took them an hour to stitch me up, and I was in pain, but it was fine. A doctor came to look at my stitches and said that they looked a bit off, but they still sent me home. With each passing day, the pain got significantly worse. But what was I supposed to know? I had never had a baby before. I thought recovery must just be a painful thing. I had been so excited to share the news with my friends and family, but because I was in so much pain, I didn't want to post about it on social media or see anyone. I just didn't feel like myself.

I felt embarrassed because I wasn't meeting my own expectations. I was like, why can't I sit on my butt? Why am I in so much pain? Why can't I walk? Why can't I do anything? I'd see all these people on social media dressed up at a coffee shop or going for walks with their babies, and it made me sad. At five days postpartum, I had an infection in my stitches. At that point, going to the bathroom was unbearable. I couldn't sit, and I had started to notice a bad smell. I went to the postnatal clinic, and they needed to cut out the infection. It was more painful than delivery or literally anything I've ever experienced. After they removed all the dead tissue, I felt a lot better. They told me that if I had waited another day or so, I would have died. I'm lucky to have found it. They put me on antibiotics, I went home, and I was pretty depressed after that. I just felt like everything sucked. I still couldn't sit on my butt, I couldn't breastfeed my baby, ***I couldn't do anything. I felt so useless and like the worst mom ever.*** I had such high expectations of myself. I was going to be that mom taking her baby out on walks. I bought a cute stroller and cute clothes, but I couldn't even sit on my butt and breastfeed my baby. It was nothing I had expected.

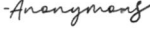

-Anonymous

No one talks about all the healing that has to happen in your body. Are you kidding me? I got muscle separation—diastasis. Also, my bladder fell. I was okay after giving birth, but then later on, it just fell. Before I had a baby, I knew there may be some stitches post labor. I knew you got swollen down there, but no one ever told me that my organs might shift or fall. I pushed for three frickin' hours during labor, and because of that, my organs got super weak. Part of my bladder fell down, and I could see it in the opening of my vagina. There was a little blob sticking out. My bladder didn't fall all the way out, but it could've happened. My doctor said if I have more kids, or if I had been a bit older, my whole bladder could have fallen out of my vagina. Now, it is a little bit uncomfortable sometimes because it is an organ that is lower than it is supposed to be, and I can feel it. I have to do a lot of Kegel exercises, which I am doing right now. I have a physical therapist, but it scares me because my bladder might be there for a long time. It could be there forever. I might need surgery eventually if I have a second or third kid. It is something I didn't expect to happen. I wish I had learned a little more about it before. I was like, can I have sex ever again? Can I use tampons again? I was freaking out. They told me, "Don't worry. You just have to keep doing your Kegel exercises." ***They don't tell you how to take care of yourself after. They send you home with a squirt bottle, then you're on your own.*** It would have been nice to have known these things in advance.

-Anonymous

Whuen you are pregnant, it's like you're this amazing vessel that's cared for and loved. Then you give birth, and you are thrown in the garbage the instant the baby comes out. You're like a piece of trash. Nobody cares about you. No one holds a door for you anymore. No one gives up a seat for you. ***You need the most care right after you have a baby.*** If you are on the verge of anything, it can push you over the edge. I had really bad postpartum anxiety, so I started going to a therapist. I'm a bit of a hypochondriac. I thought I had cancer. I couldn't even watch the news. I felt like the world was crushing me. It was really bad. I was worried about my kids all the time. Like, are they going to be killed? It wasn't rational, but at least I was able to see it. I was able to go talk to somebody. It's so nice to go to therapy. Nobody is judging you, and you can just talk about yourself and what you think. And they validate you. As a new mom, it's really nice to get some validation.

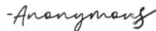

-Anonymous

I have a fifteen-year-old kid, and the older you get, the more crazy-set-in-your-ways you become. Nothing throws that out the window like a new child. When you're older, there's the good and the bad to it. What's good is that you have different resources. You can hire help. I'm obviously in a different place right now than I was fifteen years ago when we had our daughter. When I had no help, I remember being just a train wreck. I was crying every day, but this time I haven't been because we've got lots of help. But it's been physically more exhausting for me. My pregnancy was so bad: I was on bed rest for two and a half months because my rib was dislocated.

My son was breech, and his head was in my rib. I've never felt pain like that. I'm still recovering from it. I still see a chiropractor and physiotherapist because it was out of place for so long. And there's nothing they can do. His head was just jabbing my rib out of place. My doctor said, "It happens, and it's going to hurt way worse for you because you're old." When you're older, your joints are less flexible. It hurts when you're young, but for me, it was absolutely excruciating. When I think about it still, it almost brings tears to my eyes. I couldn't shower without crying. It was just (laughs) two and a half months of the most pain I've ever felt. I was gray from the pain. And you can't take anything to relieve that pain. There's nothing you can do. It was awful. Then I had to have a C-section, and the recovery from that has physically been way more difficult for me because I'm older. I would say that's been the hardest part for me. The trying to get back to normal because my whole body still hurts. I still hurt in my back, and it's almost like I'm still bruised all over—I can't put it any other way—and I think it's just because I'm older. It makes a huge difference.

Just because you can have a baby when you're older

doesn't mean you should, because it's a lot harder to recover from. And my doctor used to make jokes. She told me I was younger than her oldest patient by nine years, and I said, "Are you kidding me?" Because I was forty-seven, so her oldest patient would have been fifty-six. That's insane. I'm totally pushing the envelope, but that's crazy. People have asked if I would have another one. No way would I put my body through that again. It was just so hard.

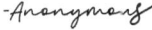

My first pregnancy was really easy, but the second one, not so much. I had a lot of discomfort, so I went to see my physio, which is where I found out I was hypotonic. I found out my pelvic floor muscles were just gripping all the time. These issues make it hard to use the bathroom, which then causes pain coupled with the added pressure of the baby. I had low-grade prolapse. So now, I was postpartum with my second child and had prolapse. It is very common. Fifty percent of women who deliver vaginally get it. Because fitness is such a big part of my life, it's been challenging. It's been challenging mentally to deal with as well because there is a lot of restriction at the beginning. You know when your mind feels ready but your body is like, this is not happening? It's really hard to stay within your capabilities when you know that you're capable of so much more. For the average person, unless they are told by a healthcare professional, they don't know about the side effects of recovery. People are told that this is just how it is: you pee a little or you experience pain when you have sex because you have had babies, so that's normal now. These effects might be super common, but they are also manageable, and in a lot of cases, you don't have to live like that. I have learned patience with my own body. You do not have to live with this kind of thing or how it affects your confidence, your mental health, and your relationships. Having a bladder prolapse makes you feel very unsexy. You feel broken. ***My vagina is broken now, and I feel unsexy.*** My marriage is a bit strained now. I don't have any desire, and it's not like I'm talking to my husband about this because it's also very embarrassing, and if I talk to him, he may find me unattractive, and I'm already uncomfortable in my postpartum body. There are so many layers to it. The hormones, everything is changing. There is so much happening at the same time, but this added level of discomfort is one of the things that we can have some control over and do something about.

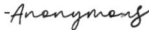
-Anonymous

What was recovery like *for you*?

_____

_____

_____

_____

_____

Write a few sentences describing your first week out of the hospital.

_____

_____

_____

_____

What were items that you absolutely needed to have when you came home from the hospital?

_____

_____

_____

_____

_____

How did these items help with your recovery?

_____

_____

_____

_____

2

NO ONE EVER TOLD ME
HOW LONELY I WOULD FEEL,
EVEN THOUGH I'M NEVER ALONE.

From postpartum isolation to pandemic isolation,
it's hard to feel like you're the only one out there.

*T**he saying "it takes a village" really puts things into perspective for those of us who don't have one.** I knew having a baby with no immediate family or grandparents close by would be hard, but my husband and I hoped that our friends would step in, at least a little bit. They were always so supportive in the past. There were so many offers of "let us know if you need anything" with no action. How am I supposed to ask my busy friend to come over and babysit so my husband and I can have a date night? We are still invited everywhere by our friends and are told that babies are welcome. But when all the plans are made after our baby's bedtime, it doesn't feel like a real invite. My friends are in different places in their lives, and they don't necessarily understand how much it would mean for them to check in on me. But it's a whole different kind of hurt when they don't ask about my baby either. Things really do change after you have a baby, but life goes on. You eventually meet other mom friends who know what you're going through, who know to check in on you, and who make concrete plans with you. You develop a new community.

-Anonymous

The most surprising thing about being a new mom is feeling trapped for so long. I've been fine with it because *I ask for help when I need to. I feel almost entitled to it because I'm postpartum.* I just need to take care of the baby. Everyone should bring me food and water and ask me what I need. It's not like that for a lot of people, but my husband really wanted to do that for me. But now he's finding it's too much. He was getting hostile about it because every two minutes I was like pass me my phone, pass me this, get me more water, get me my vitamins. Getting to a place to ask for help is huge because I almost always do everything myself. After the baby, I was naked all the time while I was pumping and breastfeeding. There is a big window in our living room. I wanted the blinds closed, and my husband kept opening them. He wouldn't listen to me. I had a total breakdown because I felt he wasn't taking care of me. I was so upset. It took that breakdown for him to actually listen, which was not really fair. But he also doesn't know how it feels. Even now, he will come home, and if I haven't changed the dishwasher, he throws a passive-aggressive fit. He says, "You should be wearing the baby and doing it." My husband gets it, but only on a certain level. Even me doing nothing is doing something. It's work. I have a premature baby, and he's gaining so much weight because of all the work I'm doing. If I was taking every opportunity to put him down and unload the dishwasher, he wouldn't be doing as well. Your contributions get forgotten because it doesn't appear like you are doing a lot because you can do it all in your pajamas. To be fair, I do feel for my husband, as he is doing everything: my bidding, the laundry, cooking dinner every night, and working. That list sounds longer than my list, but I always have to remind myself that I'm doing a lot too.

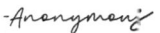

-Anonymous

I don't call family in my worst moments. If I did, they'd know this is worse than hard. Every cell in my body is screaming, and I can't let it out. I have a baby and a toddler. My marriage is suffering, and my parenting is all over the place. Everything I thought I was is now going out the window. It's just my husband and me—cleaning, feeding, soothing, and stimulating. No break, ever. I've been in the house since my baby was born in September and this is now a continuation of the isolation that has been my life since my toddler was born. This time there is no daycare, no grandparents, no girl time, no retail therapy, and no meals out. It's relative, and we are lucky. But in my relative world, most people still have nannies or just one child with two parents. ***It's all about survival, and I'm not sure who I'll wake up as each day: mom of the year or a fire-spitting, sleep-deprived Stepford wife.*** I used to like myself; at the very least, I liked who I was in relation to my family. It's all getting away from me with no end date in sight. It's just one eternal, hard-as-hell day.

—Anonymous

*T**he hardest thing about being a mom—the thing that no one told me about—is even though I have a bunch of people around me, I still feel alone sometimes.* I don't know what I'm doing. I don't know what I'm supposed to do with this infant that I'm supposed to take care of. There have been numerous times when she's been crying so much in the middle of the night, screaming in my face, and then we'll both just fall asleep. There are times when you can't do anything.

The emotional part is bigger than I expected. A lot of people talk about how their emotions just swing from one to another, and I get that. All day. I can be super happy one minute and then totally devastated the next, just because she puked on me. And I'm always crying. Like, all the time. I find days harder than nights because at least at night I can say to my husband, "I'm losing my shit. Can you go and deal with her for a minute?" But during the day, it's just me. Those are the times when it's important to have someone to talk to. I have a really huge support system—massive numbers of people who are on mat leave, as well as family members. It's nice to have those people around, but you still feel totally alone. It's a weird dynamic when you're both alone and surrounded by people. These really are the 100 days of hell. It is 100 days of you-have-no-fucking-clue-what-you're-supposed-to-be-doing-and-you're-just-trying-to-get-through-day-by-day. Nobody tells you before you have a baby that the fourth trimester is the hardest. If you knew what to expect going into it, you'd be able to mentally prepare. But it's hard to love something that's screaming in your face or puking on you every time they eat.

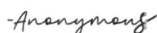
-Anonymous

O ur family and friends live across the country or overseas, and not being able to see them during the pandemic has been absolutely heartbreaking. What makes it even harder is that they haven't met our daughter who was born six and a half months ago. I'm so grateful to have such a great partner who plays many roles: best friend, husband, lover, confidant. But we have both been feeling incredibly isolated. The people who we could see, who are physically close to us, have grown less and less interested in seeing us. It's funny because these are the same friends who tell you how excited they are when you're pregnant. Working a full-time job and having no mat leave is very hard. Both my husband and I have had to work since the day our daughter was born. Because of the pandemic, we had been out of work for a few months leading up to her birth. And as soon as she was born, things started picking up again. We were struggling financially and couldn't refuse work, so we've had to say yes to everything. We work seven days a week. It's been incredibly challenging to not only take care of our daughter with zero help but also try to work forty-plus hours a week on incredibly stressful projects. We're both self-employed, so there are many nights that we've gone to bed in the middle of the night to try to make deadlines. And for me, specifically, it's been hard to focus on work during the day because my daughter feeds every two to three hours. I have a lot of anxiety about everything I do as a mom. My mom and I haven't had the easiest relationship, especially in the last couple of years, so I doubt and question everything I do with my daughter. I'm constantly worrying about everything, and it's something I didn't realize would be so gripping and omnipresent. I've also struggled with realizing that I'm a lot more sensitive and much weaker as a mom than I thought I would be. When I say weak, I mean in terms of how I deal with my emotions. When my daughter cries, I feel like my heart has been ripped out of my chest, and I will do anything in my power to console her and make her feel better. When I listen to friends and other moms speak about sleep training, I know I don't have the emotional capacity to do it. I may be making my life harder in the long run, but seeing her sad and upset bothers me so much more than I could have ever fathomed. ***Notwithstanding all the challenges and realizations, becoming a mom has filled a hole in my heart I never knew was present.*** It makes me laugh and smile more than I've ever had in my life. It makes me enjoy waking up early (something I've always despised!) and makes me want to be fully present for every single moment. It's the most beautiful feeling I've ever had.

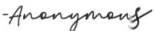

-Anonymous

*T**he hardest part of parenting is loneliness.*** I just feel so alone in my relationship. Social media makes it worse because I see people posting about going out, and I'm spending my millionth night alone at home. Yesterday, I was at my mom's house with both kids. I went to go pick up food and thought, *what if I keep driving and never come back? What if I leave my mom with both my kids?* I would never do that to my kids because of how fucked up they would be. I basically have no close friends. I have new friends that I have made along the way, but they can't remember something funny that happened growing up, or my history with my ex-boyfriends or my parents. They may know who I am, but we can't reminisce, and that contributes to feeling lonely. Everything else resets when you wake up in the morning, but the loneliness always follows you. It feels like everyone is doing something fun when I need help. I just need someone to hold my baby so I can take a shower or grab a glass of water. Everyone goes about their day, and it feels so isolating. I love to go for walks, listen to music, and dance. I used to salsa dance. There is an underground salsa community, and I love it. When I'm feeling really shitty, I think about dancing or something fun. I tell myself that a year from now I will be able to go smoke a joint, go dancing, and be free. It's my freedom.

-Anonymous

I'm a single mom. I just turned forty-three. Toward the mid to end of my thirties, I decided to freeze my eggs. My dad and I are really close, and when I made the decision, he was honest with me. He told me that this wasn't ideally what he envisioned for me. It's not what I envisioned for myself either. But I always knew I wanted kids, so I could sit around, wait, and possibly miss out, or I could do something about it. I did something about it. Nine months later, I had my baby. I was very lucky. I got pregnant the first time. I ended up having a C-section. My mom stayed with me in the hospital the first two nights. Then my parents came home with me, and they were around for the first couple days, but in the end, I told them to go. It's not like anyone else can get up at 3 a.m. and help me feed. It's the extra hand—that's what I miss. People would say their husband is not that helpful, but they still have that extra person/hand. If I had to go to the doctor, I had to bring her with. That's the hardest thing. ***I always have to get a sitter. I just figure things out because I don't have a choice.*** It's tough, it's exhausting, but I wouldn't change any of it.

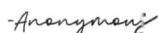

—Anonymous

The hardest part about having a newborn has been going through the isolation of postpartum during a time of global social isolation—it's almost like a double whammy. But there are positives to it. It's not so different from what I probably would have been doing. I'm home, I'm isolated, but my husband is home, which has been a huge help. I've been lucky enough that I don't want to kill him. He's very helpful. He cooks and cleans, and he's very hands on with our daughter, which is great. But we were trying to get pregnant for three years. ***We dealt with recurrent pregnancy loss and fertility-related issues for three years.*** Our families were very involved in that, and there is nothing we wanted more than to celebrate her birth with them. And we just can't do that. My family is not around. My husband's family isn't around. My best friends are not around. Introducing a new life to your family and friends over Zoom is really not ideal. We live in another country, and we had so many people coming to visit: my parents, my husband's family, my friends, and my brother. Everything is canceled. Our daughter has changed so much in three weeks. She's changing and she is growing and all I want is for my family to be a part of that. Especially after how long it took us to get here.

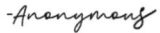

—Anonymous

Feeling lonely today? Here is a list of five things you can do when you feel lonely. Cut it out and take it with you for whenever you feel alone.

1. Call a friend. Remember phone calls? Not texts, actual calls. Your baby loves to hear the sound of your voice, but they are not old enough to know what you're saying, so it's a great time to play catch-up.

2. Join a group. Yes, mom and baby groups are often pretty awful, but it's a great way to connect with other moms with kids your age, chat about your baby, and just see other humans on the regular. Find some good online support. There are a lot of mom-focused social media accounts out there aimed at making you feel GOOD!

3. Find the one that resonates with you and don't be shy about engaging. Connection with other moms, whether in person or from afar, can help make you feel supported and seen.

4. Go to the park. First of all, fresh air always makes people feel better, but also, chances are that other moms are at the park looking to connect as well. Say hi and try to strike up conversations with other park-goers. (You can also try coffee shops or playgrounds for the same effect.)

5. Ask your friends if they know anyone who is a new mom too! Sometimes the best connections come via a friend or relative who can introduce you to someone awesome.

3

NO ONE EVER TOLD ME

HOW HARD IT WOULD BE TO

BRING MY SECOND HOME.

They tell you your heart will double and leave out
the rest . . .

I've been trying to find silver linings during the pandemic. The one that sticks out the most is my relationship with my son. He is almost two and a half, and he and I have been having a very special time for the past two months. I am there when he wakes, plays, takes a nap, and goes to bed. Pre-pandemic, I was around for about half of these events, and now there is no escape. He is my second child, and I had a hard time connecting with him for the first year of his life. I felt guilty about not spending as much time with him as I did with his older sister, not breastfeeding him as long, and leaving him with a caregiver much earlier. But if the past two years have given me anything, it's time. Lots of time. Maybe sometimes too much time, but it's given me time with him. I don't feel guilty anymore. I'm not running out the door all the time and leaving him with someone else. I finally feel that strong connection I was longing for for two and a half years. ***COVID-19 sucks, but I am fortunate for all this time with my kids that I'll probably never get back again.***

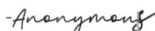

-Anonymous

I kind of feel guilty because I find it so much easier with my second child than my first. With my first, with every move she made, I'd say, "I have to call 911." I literally had never held a baby before I had one. I was scared I would drop other people's babies. I love kids, but I was really never a baby person. The first three months of my daughter's life felt like two years because I just didn't get it. With my second, it feels like it's been two days, and this time, I've just got it. I get him. I know exactly what he is about. I didn't enjoy it the first time around, and I feel guilty about that. I'm older and more mature now. I couldn't have done the two-year age gap because my first was a nightmare at that time. I'm so happy I waited. My oldest is four now. It's so important for people to know who they are and what's going to work for them. Don't be pressured—you gotta do what's good for you. I knew I couldn't handle it. There was no way I could run a business, have a partner who works like a dog, have a toddler, and then be pregnant.

—Anonymous

My husband and I always planned to have our children two years apart. As the day approached to start trying for baby number two, we were hesitant. Were we ready for another? Was it too soon? Our daughter was still so young. But we went ahead anyway and decided it would probably take us a while, as it did with our first, to conceive. Well, it turned out the due date was on baby number one's second birthday. As the day approached, I was anxious and worried. And I think going into delivery with that mindset was setting me up for failure. When they put my newborn on my chest, I cried because I instantly missed my daughter. Who was this little stranger they were handing me? I felt so unprepared for caring for two little ones. And it didn't change. The first three months were full of rage, tears, and exhaustion I didn't know existed. I was constantly overwhelmed, and I couldn't cope. I was obviously dealing with postpartum depression, but I never admitted it and never asked for help. Things improved when our son started sleeping better, but his entire first year was difficult. *I love my children and am so grateful for them, but being a mom is the hardest thing I've ever had to do.*

-Anonymous

***M*y two greatest tools after having a second baby have been perspective and experience.** Perspective: bringing home a healthy baby from the hospital is not a guarantee. Understanding this fact has been completely life altering for me. I had friends who were not able to bring their baby home from the hospital. Around the time my baby was born, there were three different cases of moms being immediately separated from their babies for weeks. So, my perspective is that if my biggest problem is that I'm tired, I'm lucky. I'm lucky that I'm home with my healthy baby, and I'm lucky to be tired because there are moms who would give anything just to be tired with their newborn. The second greatest tool has been experience. Last time, I was a wreck. I had a hard delivery, so I had a hard recovery, plus I had terrible postpartum anxiety. A lot of it is out of your control, and you're either hit with bad anxiety or depression, or you're not. I'm lucky that that didn't happen this time, but I also did the work to prepare for it. I think in certain situations, panic attacks would have come on if I had not been in therapy since having my first. I have a regular therapist, and I've had radical acceptance, which is what my therapist has taught me. Anxious moments will probably come, and they will come in waves. It's about knowing everything is a phase and that there is light at the end of the tunnel. My stitches will heal, and my gas pain will go away, and she will eventually sleep. Having that knowledge, perspective, and experience makes everything completely different the second time around. Those are the tools that have helped me survive up to this point.

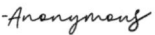

-Anonymous

I was always very open about wanting a big family. When my second son turned two, the questions began. When are you having another baby? Why aren't you pregnant yet? Little did they know, we were definitely trying for another baby; it just wasn't working in our favor. I had a miscarriage at the end of my first trimester and an ectopic pregnancy a couple of months later with a salpingectomy to remove one of my fallopian tubes. It was a difficult year. It felt like a miracle when I got pregnant four months later. We made it through the nerve-racking first trimester and the next set of questions began. Do you know the gender of the baby? How can you handle the suspense? Don't you hope it's a girl? I felt like screaming. No! Why are baby boys not enough? I never shared my experience. I felt like people asked the questions but did not want the sob story. ***To this day, whenever we go somewhere, people ask if we are going to have a fourth and "try for a girl."*** Why is having three beautiful boys not enough? I love being a mom of boys and wouldn't have it any other way.

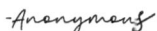

—Anonymous

I had a son, and I thought I would only have boys. And so, of course, out comes a girl! You could have knocked me over with a feather. I didn't know what to do with her, and I never thought I was going to feel that way. I thought I would feel the euphoric bliss I felt about my son. I thought I was going to feel that way times two. I thought it was going to wash over me again. Instead, I looked at her and I thought, I love you and you're my baby, but I don't know what to do with a girl. I'm going to fucking suck at this. And I proceeded to have three weeks of postpartum blues. It was really, really hard, to the point that my husband suggested I call my therapist because I was not myself. I was crying all the time. I was feeding her, I was loving her, and I was up in the night with her, but I was constantly sad. I felt sad that I was sad. And then I also had a two-year-old running around who's like totally fucked from this baby coming in. No matter how many presents you buy them, you're never going to feel like you can give yourself to them the way you did twenty-four hours prior. It blew me up, and I didn't know how to prepare for that. ***No one tells you how hard bringing the second one home is going to be.*** No one talks about it because there's so much shame around it. I just want to go back to one for an hour. I just want to give my firstborn everything, and I can't. I was already feeling like I was failing the baby because I wasn't having those skin-to-skin three-hour naps. I just remembered those cuddles with my first. I was thinking I would get to do that again, but I didn't want it as badly. I feel really lucky that I have a husband who told me to get help. I wanted to talk about it because I was struggling. I went to see my therapist. I read this list about all the things I felt shitty about. I just bawled and said, "Make me feel better. You need to fix me right now because I don't want to go home feeling this way." It took some time, but now I am fucking crazy about this little baby, and I can't imagine my family in any other shape or form. But bringing her home fucked me up big time. It was really hard, and I felt like I was failing everybody in my life. I was failing her, and I was failing my son and my husband. I didn't want to talk about it with any of my friends, and I have girlfriends. I have sister friends, and I really didn't want to admit that I was feeling blue or that it was really hard. It's never perfect. It's hard, and for anyone to say it isn't, that's bullshit. People are judgmental, and no one wants to talk about the dirty stuff—the ugly stuff.

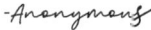

-Anonymous

Life with baby is really fucking hard right now. He's awesome, but my two-year-old is fucked. He's just so cute and so awful. I've totally sworn at him by now. I've said, "Put your fucking shoes on" multiple times. If he's being a crazy monster, I'll take him to his crib and let him be there for a little bit. I'll go upstairs in a huff, and he's over it. How do you get over it so fast? I'm still holding my grudge. He's so strong-willed and knows what he wants, but I say, "Just listen to me and do what I need you to do." He has a crazy case of mommy-itis. This morning, he was swinging the swing while the baby was in it. He was pulling the blanket off the baby, and I said, "If you do that one more time, I'm putting you in your crib." He did it and I took him upstairs, let him cool off, then I went back up. I asked him, "Why do you think that you did that?" He said, "I'm jealous." First of all, that's so sad. It's also incredible that he articulated that, but we'd been hanging out all morning. What did he want from me? What else did he need right then? ***When you're in the thick of it with two kids, there is a balancing act, and alone time is nonexistent.*** I know it passes and it gets better, but it just sucks right now.

-Anonymous

What are the differences between your firstborn and second baby? (Answers can include how they look, act, sleep, feed, or how you feel about them as a duo!)

4

NO ONE EVER TOLD ME

THAT EVERYTHING CHANGES FOR BETTER OR WORSE.

Like a good schedule or routine? That's cute. Think life postpartum is an extension of your pregnancy? Cute too. Think you've got it figured out? Even if you do, it's all about to change.

On our first night home, the baby started to cry, then I started to cry, and then my husband started to cry. I said to myself, no, you're not allowed to cry. You have to be strong for all of us right now. It's a low moment when reality kicks in and you realize life has changed for good. ***People tell you that babies change everything. But you don't understand until you're sitting with the baby and realize it's a giant blob of liability.*** I called one of my friends to ask if it's okay that I was crying. She said that I was probably just overwhelmed with love. I told her that that was not it. It was more a constant fear that the baby was going to die. I'd sit and watch the baby sleep. She has always been most comfortable on her stomach. I would lie next to her to make sure I could feel her breathing. It was terrible anxiety. I felt duped by the universe because I was surprised with the feelings I was having. Every human on the planet came from a mother who birthed them. So why are there surprises for every new mother? I should know all this stuff because it should be shared by other women who went through the exact same thing. We live in a society where we have to pay people to be our village and to help us. It's not the communal environment that it once was. I think it needs to become that way again for us to survive. You have to do the biggest job of your life with basically zero support. You feel like shit, you're wearing granny panties, and you're bleeding. You're a hot, hot mess in every way, but you're expected to bounce back. It was terrible. I was in agony. People always say that you will forget about these days, but I know I will never forget. At my six-week appointment, my doctor was talking about birth control, and I said, "We don't need to have this conversation because I'm never having another baby." I wasn't fine.

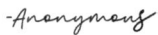
—Anonymous

L ife since having a baby has been terrible. It is the biggest game changer of game changers. I was someone who was very career oriented and focused on getting ahead. My identity was very much based on being a career woman, and I still have that part of myself. My natural self is a worker, a broker, a helper. But with my kids, I don't really want to help them. I know that sounds bad. I've been so aggravated all the time. ***I find it very frustrating with my kids. It was a weird reality check for me. I had no idea what was in store when I became a parent—I felt like I had been hit by a Mack truck.*** You have all the wrong information. I thought it was about dressing your kid in cute clothes, taking fun photos, buying a cool stroller, and getting your body back, but fuck all that shit. It is none of those things. Kids are going to shit through their nice clothes, and the stroller is a trash bin that gets banged up the second you use it because it weighs 4,000 pounds and you have to carry it everywhere. Your body is fucked no matter what you do, and most of all, those fun moments are all staged. With my first baby, I wanted to prove that I could still go out and have the same social life. I was obsessed with trying to get back into my old life. I didn't want to admit that motherhood had affected me. I wanted to be the "cool" mom but that was a total sham. I feel bad because I think that I portray that image. I think when people see me, they think I'm doing it all and I have a good grasp on it. The truth is that I don't have a good grasp on it. No one does. I'm barely sleeping, my tits are killing me all the time, I can't figure out my breast milk situation, and we are in financial debt. If it weren't for the village of people I have around me, I wouldn't be okay. I don't know how to do this by myself. So, if you think anyone is doing it better than you, they aren't.

-Anonymous

If this story sounds a bit defeated, just know that this mama then went on to have two more babies, launched (and is now running) her own business, and has faced numerous triumphs and struggles through parenting in a pandemic. Does that mean she's now doing it better than everyone else? Fuck, no. She's just doing her best—like you are, Mama. She didn't have it figured out back when we first met her, and she doesn't have it any more figured out now. That's one of the big secrets that no one tells you about being a mother: no one (and really, we mean NO ONE) has it figured out more than you. So, if you're feeling low today, just know that we've all been there.

There is always anxiety over what the night will bring. ***You go through times where the baby had a good day so you assume they are going to have a good night, and then it's total shit. Then when the day was horrible and you think they are going to be up all night, they sleep. There's no rhyme or reason, and that's what plays tricks on my brain.*** You have no idea what the next moment will bring. You've got to go with the flow, and if you're not that type of person, you have to learn quickly or it's going to be worse. I'm such a routine person. I'm a planner. I've learned to give up on certain things and control the things I can, which is nothing. It's about learning from your kid if they will go on a schedule or not and kind of feeding off their abilities. That's helped me see that the baby won't fit into my schedule, I have to fit into hers. I've been more relaxed since having a kid, which I'm shocked about. Things that would have bothered me before just don't now. Before having a baby, if I imagined her shitting or barfing on me, I would have been freaked out. Now that it's happening, I know I'm going to shower, and I know I'll be okay if she's okay. Each week she changes, and the routine changes too. She's a fairly chill kid, which has made me more easygoing because if she were higher strung, I feel like I would be higher strung. People always say she's chill because my husband and I are chill, but I think it's more the opposite. There is a lot of energy that goes back and forth. Every day I just go with whatever routine she gives me. She's had horrible days and nights, and it's not always easy. Sometimes it's just knowing that when the morning comes, a new day is here. Then after a new day, the night comes again.

-Anonymous

Because my older sister has two kids and my younger sister has one, I thought I'd be a super veteran coming into parenthood. That wasn't the case. My daughter was a big baby. There was a lot of healing, and the recovery was so painful. I've never fainted in my life, but she had just been delivered and my whole family had come to see us. I had to use the bathroom. I fainted on the floor. It's a really humbling experience. You go from this high to a really low, low. The hospital delivery room is so lovely and then the second room where they take you post-delivery is such a miserable experience. ***When you're pregnant and delivering your baby, you are Goddess Mother Earth, but after the baby comes, it's like, bye! No one gives a shit about you anymore.*** You're put in a room where your partner is shoved into a chair that maybe doesn't recline, and you're lucky if the nurses respond to you at all. My husband was on the chair holding the baby so I could rest. He closed his eyes and the nurse said he wasn't allowed to hold her because it was a liability if he fell asleep. I had to hold the baby or put her in the bassinet, and I was just in so much pain and no one gave a shit.

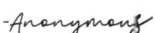

-Anonymous

I grew up in a single-parent home, and my mom worked a lot to try to make ends meet. She often had two jobs. I completely understood that she was doing the best she could, so as a child, I was super independent. Her showing love to us was working around the clock and making sure we were provided for. In many ways, that's how I am. ***My daughter and I are really close, and we have our one-on-one time, but I'm not the mom (never have been and never will be) that's at home and baking cookies.*** I get joy and value from working every day. I commend anyone who is a full-time mom, but that's just not me. I looked forward to mat leave being over. I love my daughter and I cherished that time we had together, but I find so much purpose and joy in having a career and working. Traditional roles reversed in our household during COVID-19. When we were both working from home and trying to manage our toddler, my husband was spending a lot more time with our daughter during the day. I felt a bit of guilt because of it. Should we be switching roles? Should I be with my daughter all the time because I'm the mom?

-Anonymous

We decided on names when we were pregnant. Once we found out it was a girl, we picked her name. I had a shower, and she got all these personalized gifts. I had all the guests at the shower write the baby a note, and 90 percent of them are addressed to her by name. Then we had the baby, and we filled out all the forms, like social security and the birth certificate, with the name we had chosen. We got home, a few days went by, and my husband said, "Her name isn't working for me." He just couldn't get it—it wasn't rolling off his tongue. ***So, we ended up changing her name. To this day, we have all this personalized shit for her with the wrong name.*** We didn't do a name-change announcement, so when we go to different family events or to birthday parties where we don't see people that often, they always have loot bags or gifts addressed to her wrong name.

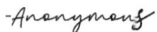

-Anonymous

S omething I am still learning is to lower expectations for myself. ***As women, we have such high expectations to be perfect in every single way.*** Part of being a mom and motherhood is riding the waves of the imperfection, and I am really trying to practice what I preach when I say that. My family life has changed in the sense that I have to be very present and aware that my eleven-year-old still needs as much attention as my seven-year-old. It's always the time management . . . like did I give enough of myself to them? In my own personal business, I promote self-care for women, and I don't think you can be a promoter if you aren't doing it as well. I get manicures every two weeks, I treat myself to a pedicure once a month, I go for walks with my girlfriends, and I have a relaxing bubble bath a few times a week. I know that I am not at my best when I am running myself ragged. I have always allowed myself to have that time. I didn't make time for self-care with my first two kids. I was mentally and physically exhausted. I just recognized over a lot of years and healing that you need to take care of yourself.

-Anonymous

*N*o one ever told me about the conflicting information you get as a parent. Someone says do A, B, C, D, and then you read something five seconds later that says the exact opposite. I didn't realize how combative and judgmental this whole baby world could be. If you're doing something different than a group is, then you are just a terrible mother—or at least that's how it makes me feel. "Do what works for you" is a piece of advice that I've gotten a lot. Now I understand what it means. At the time I didn't, because it was my first child and I had no clue. But doing what works for you makes sense now because there are so many conflicting ideas and approaches.

How to put a baby to sleep has been one of the things that I have struggled with. I'm working with an amazing sleep consultant, but at the same time, I'm a bit of a wimp, and I'm having a hard time sticking to the program. My instinct is to run in there and grab my baby and make sure she is okay. We did research before starting the sleep-training journey. One side says the baby is fine and crying it out isn't harmful. That made me feel so much better, but then I would read message boards with parents who shame by saying, "How dare you let the baby cry it out." I'm in the middle and I want to do what feels right. If it takes a bit from column A and from column B, then maybe that's fine because I don't need to spend time thinking whether I'm terrible for doing it this way.

It came down to what was best for me because I was starting to lose myself. I felt myself falling into depression and constant sadness. I decided to make some changes because I didn't want to feel like that. I want to enjoy my daughter and I want her to be happy. I want her to sleep through the night, and we are going to get there. We are going to do it on our own terms and in a way that will incorporate both groups of thought. I need to make it better because when I'm better, she is better. I deal with anxiety, and I have been doing great for years, but it's funny how this whole journey has brought bits of it back. Once I realized that it was all brewing to the surface, that's when I was like, okay we can't go back there again. I don't want my time with my daughter to be filled with anxiety.

-Anonymous

I present myself as pretty chill, but I'm actually secretly really type A. I want everything to be perfect and structured. I'm also very anxious about safety stuff. Knowing that I'm like that, I try and take a step back and also let them be babies. I'm trying to find that balance. I was a very scheduled person. Like, nap has to be every three hours. I was that person. ***There is so much information and there is so much contradicting information that I never knew what to do.*** I would read something, and it would say you should start sleep training them at twelve weeks and they should be in a crib, and then I would read something else that would say just let it happen. That was a little bit challenging. I'm still a bit more rigid, but I'm trying to let things go. I think having a baby made my anxiety a bit worse, though. Initially, I thought it would be easy. Like, he would just sleep from this time to this time, but then he'd wake up unexpectedly and I would be so flustered. I was more anxious because he didn't follow what I wanted. I had to really let that go, which wasn't easy at all. That was one of the hardest things. I wanted to do certain things, and I needed him to fit into my schedule. That's not how babies work, and it really sucks.

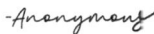

-Anonymous

Write down your current schedule. Include everything you do in a day with your baby. Then come back in a month or two and write it all down again.

_____

_____

_____

_____

_____

_____

_____

_____

_____

_____

_____

_____

_____

_____

_____

_____

_____

_____

What's changed?

_____

_____

_____

_____

_____

5

NO ONE EVER TOLD ME
HOW TRIGGERING EVERYTHING
COULD BE AS A NEW PARENT.

Hate your mom? Your MIL? Your Instagram feed?
Your traditions? Hate it all? Read on …

My husband is Jewish and I'm not. We originally were not going to circumcise the baby because we aren't religious, and it was not something we wanted to do. And then his parents conveyed why it was very culturally important to them. There was a lot of back-and-forth. We felt uncomfortable doing a religious ceremony for something we don't practice. My family didn't push for a baptism, even though it's common in my family. Strangely, all the boys in my family are circumcised even though we are not Jewish. I think in the '80s when we were all born, circumcision was thought to be healthier or cleaner. In Canada, more people are uncircumcised than circumcised. I did a lot of research; I wanted to prepare myself to have this discussion. My fear about a circumcision is that you are getting rid of thousands and thousands of nerves. And as a sex-positive parent, I don't want to—for literally no reason besides a religion that I don't believe in— deny him pleasure for the sake of doing something for someone else. But we ultimately decided to have a circumcision at a hospital with the head of urology who also happens to be a mohel. It doesn't count as a religious service, but it feels like a compromise with his family. We have an appointment, and I'm really nervous about it because it's a tiny baby. ***So many of my friends' kids have been circumcised, and everyone says the same thing—it's horrible.*** Neither of us are thrilled about it.

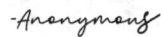

-Anonymous

N o one ever told me how many people would comment on my postpartum body. I come from an immigrant family, and I was the first one born in Canada. We have a huge extended family and every adult, specifically the women, had something to say about what others' bodies looked like: "Oh, you look really good—you look really skinny." Then the next time they would say, "Oh, you've gained some weight; that dress is really unflattering." They would say really specific things to us about our bodies. I grew up like that from the time I was a little kid. Everything was based on how I looked. They never asked about anything else, and so that's just how I thought about body image.

When I became pregnant, my mom was so excited because it was her first grandchild, but I was a vessel. I was this beautiful vessel giving birth to her coveted granddaughter, so obviously, when my daughter was born, my mom didn't care about me anymore. Then the comments started again. She would tell me that I don't need to take care of myself because I'm a mom now or I would complain about my body and she would say, "Yeah, you've gained a lot of weight." ***When I lost the baby weight, she would still make comments including, "Your arms still look fat."*** She would comment on parts of my body every time I would see her, and it would make me feel terrible.

It's definitely a cultural thing: she just says stuff and is very blunt. She does it without any prompting, and it's just the way she talks. I have tried to stand up for myself, but it's so hard. My husband is white, and so sometimes he will jump in, but it doesn't stop. It's something I've struggled with my whole life, and I feel like no matter what I've done with my body, she's going to say something. So, I am trying hard not to do that to my daughter. I want to break that cycle, but it's so ingrained in me.

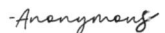
-Anonymous

I had my baby in Taiwan so I could be with my family. ***I was looked at funny because I left the house with my baby, and in Chinese/Taiwanese culture, people don't really bring their kids out until a month after the baby is born.*** I was so happy when I went to apply for the baby's passport, because I had an excuse to leave the house. It was so nice to just be out and be doing something other than breastfeeding and changing diapers. We were walking with the baby at the park and this woman closely followed me and said, "Oh wow, your baby looks so small. How old is she?" When I said three weeks, she told me I shouldn't have my baby outside because it's really windy. So many people said that I shouldn't be out because of the weather. It was not cold at all—it was 25°C. I got into arguments with my mom over it. She actually told me that if I didn't rest properly that my health would be ruined for life. That's what people believe. You're also not supposed to drink anything cold. My mom was adamant about it. When I came home from the hospital, I ate healthfully. I drank bone broth and things that help stimulate breast milk production, but I wasn't going out to go eat bird's nest or shark fin soup. Technically speaking, you are not supposed to wash your hair for forty days, but then again, that was from the old days when there were no hair dryers or heaters. When it's cold outside, they don't want you to wet your hair and get a chill. I was so hot all the time, I was not about to put a jacket on. I was not going to do anything that would make me uncomfortable. It was hard for my partner and me because we didn't understand the whole culture and the reasons for these decisions. I tried to ask, but it seemed like a tradition that was passed on that no one really understood. I don't really know what to believe.

-Anonymous

I always imagined what it would feel like to have a baby. The physical stuff for sure, but I spent a lot of time imagining the emotional stuff too. I never worried that I wouldn't attach to my baby. At the time I had her, my friend also just had a baby, and she talked about being overwhelmed with love. I was not there. I loved this baby, but I didn't feel an overwhelming sense of love. It felt scarier and more of a liability than love. Love wasn't the feeling that came first or top of mind. I don't think I fully, deeply became obsessed with her for a while. When I was pregnant, I would always look up newborn hashtags on Instagram and see people in the hospital holding their new babies. They always looked so in love, but I wondered if it was all a lie. But also, fuck you all. Did a hairdresser come to the hospital, wash your hair, and blow dry it? I don't understand. My friend has a picture of her post-delivery holding her baby, and her hair is blown out and she looks beautiful. So, not only was I expecting to just be head over heels in love with my baby, I was also expecting to look beautiful. I just thought I would be gorgeous and in love. Instead, I felt scared of this baby and the pictures are all of me with a triple chin, a rat's nest of hair in a bun, and the hospital gown falling off me. ***I feel like we get so tripped up about what is expected because of social media. Everybody lied to me. It felt like everyone was tricking me.***

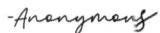

-Anonymous

M*y mother-in-law is funny. My husband is forty-two, and she still sees him as her baby who she needs to take care of.* I dread going to her house for dinner. On the one hand, I love it because she is an amazing cook and sends us home with lots of food, but when we get there, it's very unrelaxing for me. My husband grew up in that house, so he's fully comfortable, and he can just chill on the couch. But I can't relax. Their house is massive, and it's not fully baby-proofed. Every time I go there, I find a miscellaneous pill in the carpet. They have this stupid rocking horse that neighs, but the neigh was dying so they had to change the battery. I'm super anxious about safety things, especially about batteries. My husband was on the couch watching the baseball game, and his mom busted out all these batteries on the ground. She picked up a small watch battery and said, "Where did this come from?" Oh, my God. I started to sweat, and I threw pillows at my husband to get his attention. In the meantime, his mom found another battery in the carpet. Whenever we go there, she is always doting on my husband while the kids are running around and I'm chasing them. It's not fun for me. I'd rather say no to a great dinner and leftovers because I spend the whole time chasing the kids around. It's just that crazy social dynamic. Why should only the mother or the female need to fill that role?

-Anonymous

*T**he first time doing anything with a baby is rough.**
The first time I left the house with her to go to the mall, it was February, and it was awful. Even just packing the car. I probably went to and from the car four times because of forgetting things. You bring way too much stuff the first time—it's an overload of crap. And then the second time you have less, the third time you have less, and the fourth time you have less. Then the fifth time they shit themselves, and you wish you had that extra change of clothes. When I got to the mall, I felt like everyone was staring at me. Judging me—like hardcore judgments. I felt like I was carrying my daughter wrong and someone was going to say something and it would be internalized forever. Or her leg was sticking out of her carrier the wrong way and I was going to break her. It's all because of other people's opinions that aren't even being said; they're just being felt. I felt their judgments. I felt like a mom impostor. Like it's not my baby and I have no fucking clue who this thing is that I'm taking care of."

-Anonymous

S omeone I knew who had a baby around the same time as me was posting selfies. I can't even wash my face, let alone take a picture and post it online. And everything in our house is a disaster. There's stuff everywhere. I just felt so awful, and then the next thing I saw was a live video from another friend who just had a baby and she's perfect: makeup done, hair done, and her baby's sleeping. She was doing an Instagram Live about bath salts, and I wondered how she did it. How was she able to put herself together? At this point, I can't even answer my text messages, and I feel helpless. ***People are totally doing this amazing job on social media, and I feel so alone.*** I know I have a good group of supporters, but I really feel alone. You lose your identity in it. It's like all of a sudden, you don't know who you are. You don't know it when you have your first baby. No one tells you about this darkness thing and how you will feel. I always wanted two kids, but I never thought I'd be in the place of not wanting another because of being so in it. It's so dark that I can never imagine going through it again. There are days when I feel like I've got it, and then days when I'm not okay.

-Anonymous

My mother has always been difficult, but her behavior escalated when I got pregnant. It was all about her being a grandparent and wanting me to need her, ask for advice, and defer to her on decisions and parenting. She even called me her incubator and sulked when I didn't talk to her before anyone else. If I said anything or parented differently than the way she raised me, she would cry or stop speaking to me or call me uptight and ungrateful. ***It felt like I had to choose between what I believed in and wanted for my kids and doing things my mom's way to avoid her rejecting and attacking me.*** She refuses to visit or help because she thinks I should visit her and make an effort as her daughter. I've ruined her chance to be a grandmother, apparently. It's been a lesson in boundaries—learning to stand in my own truth with feeding, sleeping, gentle parenting, and how I deserve to be treated. I would never have stood up for myself if it wasn't for my children. Now I see how they look to me for what is right and what is not. I have been brave enough to say no more often for them. I have learned to stand up for myself so that one day they can too.

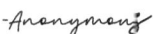
-Anonymous

My mom and my mother-in-law are both helping, but then they always put in their two cents. Every day my mother-in-law calls me and asks me if I have done this or done that. Oh, my God. It's nice to get the help, but it's a little too much. Everyone says I'm so lucky, but it's stressful too. ***My mother-in-law lives right across the street, so every time I need her she is able to come, but sometimes it is too much help and too much information.*** I see my mom once a week. You want the help, but sometimes it is too much help. I love having my mother-in-law so close, because anytime I need something last minute or have a doctor's appointment, I have her come over and watch the baby, but whenever she is here, she has lots of different ideas. Times have changed since thirty years ago when she had her son. For example, salt. I don't want to give my baby anything salty when I start solids, and she keeps telling me when I start to feed the baby I should cook with salt and, you know, how do I fight that?

-Anonymous

What are some things that trigger you? Write them down and then pick one. How can you help yourself with this trigger? OR How can you give yourself permission to let it go?

If you've got one, share your best "shit my mother-in-law says."

We'll start: "My mother-in-law asked how much weight I had lost while I was in the delivery room."

6

NO ONE EVER TOLD ME
ABOUT THE BOUNCE BACK.

FUCK THE BOUNCE BACK.

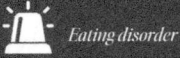 *Eating disorder*

I went into labor, fully expecting to deliver vaginally. The alternative didn't occur to me, likely because my pregnancy—though long awaited after eighteen months of trying—was easy. I mean, growing a human isn't easy, but I didn't have most of the common issues pregnant women face, and I was pretty enamored over the whole experience. So, when my water broke on my due date, the last thing I expected was to end the journey with a belly birth. And since that day I've struggled with what that meant and now means to me. Did I fail? Did I do something wrong? Now my body has this scar and this ridge of tissue above my pelvic bone that I am really struggling to accept. I don't want it. Don't want to look at it. Don't want to touch it. And I certainly don't want anyone else touching it. Before being pregnant, I felt pretty comfortable in my body. I was proud of how strong it was and all the things it could do. And though it took a bit of work to get out of my head and into my body, I could feel attractive and sexy regularly. Now, I question everything. Is my body strong? How could it be if it failed in the one thing I assumed it would do? If I think that this scar is unlovable, how can my partner love it?

How can I feel worthy of love and touch and desire when I don't feel confident in my body anymore? And how can I shut off these fucking thoughts and just be in my body and be intimate with him again? I've spent the majority of my postpartum journey with absolutely zero sex drive. It only came back just before my period did. I'm relieved it did, but I still haven't figured out how to carve out time in days that are so long and demanding mentally and physically to find that closeness. That sexiness. That desire. And I'm so scared that he'll give up on me. You just don't know what you're signing up for when you start your pregnancy journey, do you?

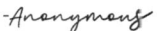
-Anonymous

I was at my thinnest when I got pregnant. I was a bridesmaid for my cousin's wedding, so I was working hard and eating really well. Not only was I at a good weight, I was also toned and felt really good. And then we started trying and I got pregnant right away. I gained seventy pounds. My OB was okay with it because I was healthy, but I felt so big. I couldn't walk properly, people had to help me stand up, and my feet and hips hurt. I wasn't used to carrying all that weight. I didn't feel good, and I wanted her out because I worked hard to be an optimal weight. ***I hate the bounce back because it's BS and unfair to everyone with different body types.*** I love my mom friends, but none of them gained as much weight as I did, and many of them were able to lose the baby weight immediately after giving birth. I managed to lose about fifty pounds. It was so hard, and it seemed like no one else had to. It's like a test: you can put in all the work and do all the studying, but you can still do badly compared to someone who studied a bit less or not at all. I've had body image issues my whole life. I've had an eating disorder, and I've gained lots of weight and lost lots of weight. It's an unrealistic ideal. I don't mind having a bit of extra weight, but I don't fit into my clothes. I just want to feel okay in the clothes that I like. Right now, I'm not there; right now, I hate everything. I know my body did this amazing thing. I grew and pushed out a baby, but I just want my old body back. No one validates this feeling. They always say, "It's okay" or "You look great." It's never an actual conversation about feeling shitty about myself.

—Anonymous

I have always looked at my body critically. After I had my daughter, I was in a group to motivate me to work out more and eat better. We were always sending each other selfies about the changes in our bodies, and I felt good about it at the time. But I was always looking at my body and thinking that my stomach could be tighter, I could get some more muscle, my arms aren't defined, and my thighs are too jiggly. *I was always trying to be more toned, but my mentality changed when I started feeding my kid solids. Now with her in mind, I am trying to be more focused on food nourishing us and not trying to aim for that next little change.* It's not even on my mind anymore, and what I ended up doing is that I changed my Instagram grid and started following a lot of fat-positive influencers and people with diverse body types. I realized that seeing thin women in bikinis and fitness influencers was giving me negative points of comparison. By having a range of bodies on my grid, it gives me perspective on how people look different. It's been a big shift for me.

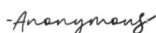
-Anonymous

Before having my own babies, I taught pre- and postnatal yoga for five years. My students taught me so much about their journey toward motherhood. They shared their birth stories and postpartum struggles and triumphs. I never paid attention to the weight gain and loss aspect of pregnancy and motherhood. My classes were aimed at supporting my students' mental, emotional, and physical health. The "bounce back," in my humble opinion, is a myth. A horrible and unrealistic standard perpetuated by North American society that has become obsessed with perfection. Is perfection your pre-pregnancy body? To some, yes . . . and that is okay. To others (a.k.a. me!), there are things on the self-care to-do list that don't involve excessive planking, cardio, weights, etc. My children are six, five, and two. I had three C-sections. My priority as a new mom was never to flatten out my tummy. I embrace my mom pouch because it reminds me of how insanely amazing our bodies are. Part of my mental health is reminding myself that it is okay my tummy has some bulge and excess skin. My body is miraculous, down to every last wrinkle and roll. I have earned the right to be happy and secure with how my physical appearance is today. Fuck the bounce back. ***It's unfair to assume a woman is not happy until she sheds her baby weight.*** All you can do is trust the process, find gratitude in the body you have, and remind yourself every day that you are beautiful and sexy just the way you are.

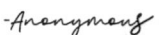

-Anonymous

I was buying a lot of clothes online to figure out my new body. It's changed since having a third. I'm like a barrel now. Pants don't fit my waist, and shirts are too tight. I just wanted to buy new stuff, and I went bananas. I'm not happy with my body, and I'm buying shit from all over the internet. I'm looking at the hottest chicks alive for inspiration, and I'm like, why are you doing that to yourself? You have to be kind to yourself. Don't buy stuff like that. At this time, three weeks out from having a third, don't buy a crop top. You just had a baby. All the clothes in my closet are maternity or from before when I was working out and in better shape—there's no in-between. My size small jeans and my maternity clothes are right there in front of me, and I wonder, where am I now? Where do I fit now? I know it's still early, but you think everything should be back to normal. ***I want my body back. I want my hair to not constantly be in this fucking scrunchie. I want to go back to normal.*** Will I get back to that? Will I actually be normal? Probably not.

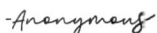

-Anonymous

I take him to Stroller Fit where every other baby is silent. He screams the whole time. And the moms are all wearing really nice workout clothes. I don't know how their bellies look the way they do. I'm in my nursing bra, pulling my boob out, while they're all doing a full forty-five-minute workout. And I'm just sitting there in the shade watching them. I thought I had such an easy child, but there's literally twenty-five people there all dressed perfectly and working out with completely silent babies. I don't know if the moms give them drugs before they go to class, but I stopped going because I did maybe five minutes of exercise. Should I give my kid a Benadryl and then go? It's not really real—for me at least. A mom I know gets her hair done and she looks so gorgeous. Her baby is six weeks younger than mine, and I'm like, what the fuck are you doing? I see her in jeans and a blowout. I feel like one of those moms on TV that's looking around and everyone is perfect. ***Sometimes I look on Instagram and I'm upset that people seem to juggle it all so well.***

—Anonymous

My mother-in-law asked me how much weight I had lost right after I delivered. Basically, they had just taken the IV out of my arm. It made me realize that society places so much pressure on moms. My mother-in-law isn't vain. She's an amazing, humble woman. It's just how society has trained us to think. These are the questions that her mom asked her, and it's the messages that are put out there in the media. ***There's all this pressure to change your appearance and bounce back.*** No one tells you that those comments, every single one of them, is going to scar. When someone comments about what you look like or how you're breastfeeding, they don't see that behind the scenes, you're drowning inside. We wear this body armor every single day, and you have to brush things off. You don't have a choice. You can't melt down every time. People make comments in every interaction about something, but when you're so lost in yourself, it hurts so much more.

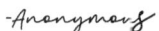
-Anonymous

I credit women who look in the mirror and want to see their stomach. When it is a hard ball, you just accept it. But when the baby comes out, you're enormous and flabby. I don't look in the mirror. I will get a side view and still hate it. My eating disorder is years gone, way behind me. And the body image stuff is better, but I always like to look and dress a certain way. The most awful part of the weight gain and how I look postpartum is that it brings me back to what I hated most about myself. Even during my pregnancy, people said, "You are beautiful," "You look amazing," "You're not fat." And I said, "No, I'm fat." I never wanted to take pictures. It's the worst thing that could happen to someone like me because of my history with an eating disorder. My children are the biggest blessing, and I'm ecstatic to have beautiful, healthy children, but it's just not easy for me. I don't want to go out; I don't feel good. I don't know if it affects me in the way that I starve myself to get back down to the pre-birth weight, but I put a lot of pressure on myself to snap right back into perfection—and it doesn't work that way. ***The fourth trimester is so layered. You have a newborn, you're not sleeping, you're not eating properly, and no one talks about your body image.***

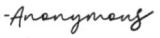
-Anonymous

Name five things that are amazing about your body. Cut out this page and tape it to your mirror so you remember when you're feeling like shit.

7

NO ONE EVER TOLD ME

HOW DIFFICULT
BREASTFEEDING WOULD BE.

By bottle or breast, either is best.

After the hospital, we were home at 5 a.m. and the midwife was coming back to check on us at 7 p.m., so we had to kind of figure out breastfeeding ourselves. Somehow, it seemed to work. The latch looked really good, and our son gained back his birth weight in four days. I had no problems with supply, and everything was great for two weeks. And then the screaming started. It was like torture for him when I nursed. I kept going back to the midwife and she said everything looked fine. I would nurse at night, and he would scream for an hour until he fell asleep. He would sleep for half an hour, wake up, and then we'd do the whole dance again. I went to a girlfriend's house, one who had had a baby a week later than I did, and I watched her breastfeed. The baby fed for fifteen minutes, burped, fed on the other side, and then went to sleep. That was not happening with my baby. I kept going back to the midwife who thought everything looked great. He was gaining weight, so we were not concerned from that perspective, but it got to the point where I couldn't breastfeed. I was so embarrassed by the screaming, and I had no way of settling him. I wasn't sleeping at all, and my husband's career was busier than ever. He would leave at 7 a.m. and come back at 7 p.m., and he worked all weekend. At three weeks postpartum, I hit rock bottom. I was so exhausted and depressed. I asked him if he could take a feeding shift on the weekend. The first time we did that, the baby didn't scream at all. He drank the bottle, burped, then fell asleep. I had changed my whole diet. I wasn't drinking coffee, I wasn't eating cheese, I wasn't doing anything because I thought the whole issue was my milk, but he took a bottle of pumped milk no problem. It was lovely. I feel like once he had a bottle, he had no interest in the boob. On the weekend, he would do bottles and I kept nursing. ***Everyone kept saying*** *everything was fine and I was like, what is going on? I have the milk, I have the position, I have the latch, everything is fine, but something isn't fine.* Then it turned into a lot of social isolation. I would try to nurse in public. One time I was at the grocery store, and he just wailed. There was this group of high school kids eating their lunch and they were like, get your shit together, woman! At eight weeks, we got a night nurse, and she wanted to try a bottle of formula. He drank it and went to sleep for five hours. Then I was doing a bottle of formula each night, and he slept through the night at three months, whereas he wouldn't sleep more than two hours before the formula. I started providing formula at night while still nursing during the day. He wasn't screaming as much, but he wasn't eating, so I nursed every forty minutes. He couldn't sleep because he was constantly hungry, so I decided to try a whole day of just bottles of breastmilk. It was the best day we'd ever had together. He was happy.

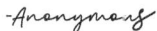
-Anonymous

It's my first baby so it's a bit of shell shock because everything has changed. There's not one thing I recognize from my life. I said to my sister who has two kids, "Why does everyone focus on all the wrong things?" ***No one told me about the real hard things like breastfeeding and the issues around feeding.*** Feeding is such a huge thing, and everyone is focused around having the right crib or clothes—all the cute stuff. I was panicking because I didn't know what to do about bottles. Like what bottles do you use? It's so overwhelming, and breastfeeding is not intuitive. I was waiting for my milk to come in at the hospital. They were giving my baby formula, and nobody told me I had other options. We had to get a lactation consultant to come to the house because I was a mess. Why did no one tell me this? I was about to get mastitis, and I didn't know what to do. Because when you're sleep deprived, you're not going to be able to do research. So, it was interesting because it was the things I never would have expected that I found the hardest.

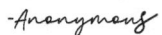
-Anonymous

I had no idea how much trouble breastfeeding would be. You would think it is something that comes naturally to babies. But it doesn't happen like that. I pump when the baby naps because I can't breastfeed him. It's exhausting. I pump three times during the day, but it's a lot to even find the time to do that. I try to use my organizational skills to make it happen—I work as a project manager. He naps thirty minutes to the dot, and that's exactly how long I need to pump. He wakes up the second I stop washing all the pump parts. I have the pump that you can walk around with, so while I'm pumping, I do dishes and laundry. Thank God I have some experience managing my time because I don't know how else I would get by. It's exhausting, and that is something nobody tells you. They tell you having kids is so amazing and beautiful. They tell you that you are going to love your time on mat leave. Well, yeah, there are days when I am super happy, but there are days when everything is too much. Sometimes I want my life back. **Nobody tells you that your life changes. I am outgoing, a social butterfly, always going out and meeting new people. Now it is so different; I can't leave my house. I need to stay home to pump for the baby.** I am stuck. It's a completely different life. It's not a bad life. I love my baby, but it is a different life now.

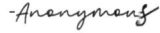

-Anonymous

My expectations have changed. I knew I was probably going to formula feed this baby because I have three kids under three and I can't do it all. With my first kid, I said I was never giving formula, but who even cares? And sometimes even if you do care, circumstance makes you change your priorities . . . or you give yourself a bit more grace when you're not trying to be the best parent in the world. This time I couldn't care less, and I'm good with it. I have no expectations of myself. But the amount of pushback I've had from people about formula is crazy. They ask me all the time why I'm formula feeding. It doesn't bother me, but if I was in a different headspace, it would really get to me. In the hospital, no one at any point asked me if I was formula feeding, if I had a bottle on me, if I needed to know anything about how much to make up or give her. I remember asking how much to give a newborn, but no one would answer me. I didn't get a straight answer. It wasn't set up to support a mom who had made the decision to formula feed. ***You have to find ways to be able to enjoy it, and for me, that's formula feeding, bottle feeding, whatever I can do to make everything manageable.***

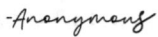

-Anonymous

***I**'m constantly filled with mom guilt because I didn't breastfeed.* I fed my son for a month, and I fed my newborn for four days because she needs a happy mom, and breastfeeding did not make me happy. It was really hard. And that's something they don't tell you: how hard breastfeeding actually is. It's a full career, and I credit every mother who breastfeeds. Choosing not to breastfeed can eat at you for no other reason than societal pressure. I internally felt okay giving my baby formula, but the outside world puts such shame over it. Even at my doctor's office when they ask if I'm breastfeeding or using formula, I just want to cover my face when saying that she's on formula.

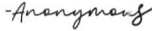

-Anonymous

Breastfeeding is one of the biggest challenges. At the very beginning, they say you need to exclusively breastfeed. I gave birth at the hospital and there was a great breastfeeding clinic the morning after I had my baby. But I was so out of it that I couldn't keep my eyes open. I couldn't get anything out of it. ***They shame you if you don't breastfeed.*** I had such a hard time. I was barely getting a drop out, and when I got home, I could hardly feed her. No one told me I should have some formula. I wasn't given any alternatives. No one ever told me it was going to be that difficult. I saved every last drop of the colostrum, but it just wasn't enough to feed her. That was overwhelming. I went to the family doctor for the post-delivery checkup. The baby had lost way more than 10 percent of her weight, so they sent us to the hospital where we rushed to see the lactation consultant. They weighed her and gave her a bottle of formula after they had basically been shaming me to not use formula. Obviously, that is what she needed. She was just thirsty and hungry. They gave me some tips, and I got a nipple shield because I have really flat nipples. The baby was having difficulty latching properly. I didn't really know that was a thing. Things were better once I got the shield. It actually works like a charm, and I still use it. It's really good because I don't have any blistering or chapping on my nipples. I do a combination of that and bottle feeding, which gives so much flexibility. My husband can feed her, we can go outside, and I'm not stressing about having to pull out my boob in the middle of winter. I probably breastfeed her twice a day, and the rest is bottle. I had some blocked ducts, which were really painful. No one talks about that. It opened up a conversation with my mom and her girlfriends. They started talking about their experiences breastfeeding because I brought up all these bad stories. It got them to admit that they also had bad experiences because no one really talks about it.

-Anonymous

People stare at me all the time when I'm breastfeeding in public. I went to the grocery store the second week after I gave birth. I like going to get groceries. I'm not one to order online. I like to physically pick my apples and stuff. My mom came with me. We brought the stroller, and we had a cart. My son (obviously) lost it in the grocery store the second we got there. It already took us two hours to get there because he was screaming in the car, and I had to take him out, feed him, and burp him. So I was feeding him around the store, walking with my cover on, and everyone was staring at me. You do it where you have to do it. Don't stare at me while I'm humiliatingly trying to walk around the aisles feeding my child. My mom was pushing the stroller and the cart at the same time, and we were just a hot mess. It happened again the other day. After we paid at the cash, I was taking him off my boob and it was hanging out. I didn't even feel it. You know how your boobs get numb? And my boob was just hanging out. My mom was with me again and she said the favorite part of her day was when I flashed everyone at the grocery store. Stuff like that happens to me all the time. ***I constantly feel like a hot mess because my boobs are always hanging out.***

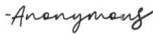

-Anonymous

No one gave me the memo on nursing. I was encouraged to nurse, and it was pretty easy because I make a lot of milk. But boy, did my boobs go through the ringer. ***No one ever talks about all the shit that comes with breastfeeding.*** I felt like I had blocked milk ducts every other day. I was so engorged, and I didn't know how to manage it. I had to get super resourceful about how to get that milk out so that I wouldn't have blocked ducts all the time. It was crazy what I had to go through. There was one time that I had an insane blocked duct. It was next level pain, and I couldn't get it out. I did all the bullshit in the shower, I did the bath, I massaged it, I did the self-expressing. Nothing worked. So, I made my husband suck my boob. He cleared my milk. I was desperate. I couldn't explain to the baby how to suck it. I told my husband, "Honey, you're going to need to do this for me." I was literally on all fours over him, and I'm pretty sure he was turned on. He got it out. I always knew we loved each other and there was a lot of love in our relationship, but that moment right then, that was LOVE.

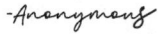

-Anonymous

O nce we were out of the delivery room, they abandoned me, my baby, and my husband in a semi-private room. I remember my heart dropping. I went from receiving all this great care to absolutely nothing. I just wanted to cry. I was so terrified. The nurse came and wanted the baby to feed right away. She was so rough with me as she was grabbing my boobs. It was humiliating. They are squeezing you like a cow and trying to do all this stuff while you are still in shock from having a baby. My son didn't latch then, and he never really did after. That was the worst part. It would be great if he could breastfeed, but it was such a traumatic experience to get shamed because I couldn't figure it out properly. There were some nurses who would try to help me, and then there were others who would just take my breast and shove it in his mouth. It was so violent and terrible. We were in the hospital for two days and we saw a couple of lactation consultants. Finally, we found out that I had an extremely low milk supply, so when he did latch, he didn't really get anything. We kept trying to breastfeed for a while. We went to numerous lactation consultants, and most of them shamed me for not being able to breastfeed properly. Even though I knew in my heart that he just needed to eat, I almost needed them to say it was okay to give him formula. The last consultant said that formula was the worst thing I could give my baby. And I thought: this is my only option? Fuck you. That was the worst part of my whole experience. ***Breastfeeding was something I really wanted to do, but I got shamed for not being able to.*** Now he is on formula. He's going to eat McDonald's one day, so I think formula is OKAY.

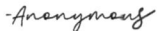
-Anonymous

I took my son to the hospital three days postpartum because they didn't take his blood properly. They encouraged me to feed him while they took the blood. I couldn't feed him. The lactation consultant described my breasts as rock-hard soccer balls. I had planned to be at a work event that day. In some delusional, fucked up world, I thought I would be able to attend an event and give a speech because I had no idea I would be a total disaster. I was getting messages from my colleagues about the event, and I was sitting there in the hospital bawling my eyes out because I couldn't feed my child. It was so eye-opening for me. ***I can do so many things, but breastfeeding was the hardest emotional and physical thing I've ever had to do. And it's the most natural thing—so they say.***

-Anonymous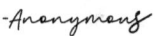

I chose to _____
(feed by breast, bottle, exclusive pumping, and/or a combination of
the two) and here is what I loved about it:

_____

_____

_____

_____

_____

_____

_____

_____

_____

_____

_____

_____

_____

_____

_____

_____

_____

_____

_____

_____

_____

_____

_____

_____

_____

_____

8

NO ONE EVER TOLD ME
HOW HARD HAVING A BABY IS
ON YOUR RELATIONSHIP.

The best birth control in the universe.

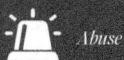 *Abuse*

Mental illness can wreak havoc on a relationship. When I got pregnant, my husband's mental illness got much worse. He was barely present during the pregnancy, but I kept hoping he'd step up. After a grueling twenty-eight-hour induced labor and four hours of pushing, I was more mentally and physically drained than I've ever been in my life. My son had low blood sugar and was jaundiced and severely tongue-tied, and my husband's primary concern was making sure he went home to sleep. I felt intense relief when my brother stayed the night to help monitor my son in the incubator. My husband and I fought in the hospital about my family being around to help. He wanted to be the one engaging with the baby, but he only took action when it suited him.

The first night home from the hospital, I had an episode where I shook uncontrollably and almost dropped the baby. I didn't call for my husband. I called for my dad, who wrapped me in blankets and gave my son a bottle so I could rest. I was delirious for the first two weeks with a bad bladder infection. I struggled with breastfeeding—it was torture and took everything I had. And in the midst of all this, there was fight after fight. My husband was completely focused on his own experience and wasn't making room for mine. He slept in another room to get rest and would sleep through alarm after alarm to take the baby before work. Then he'd struggle with the baby and wake me to salvage things. I started to think that having my husband there was harder work than doing it alone. Then, the lockdowns started. I was six weeks postpartum with a husband completely unable to cope with himself, let alone his newborn and wife. All my support—my doula, cleaning lady, family visits—were being stripped away. I was so incredibly alone. Then one morning my husband slept through another alarm to wake up with the baby. I hadn't slept for more than thirty-minute stretches all night, all with the baby in my arms. Sometime later, he woke up and took the baby for a bit. Finally, sleep. He barged in, turned on the lights, and paced back and forth at the foot of the bed yelling. His anger filled the room and his delusions blinded him to what was in front of him. I sat up bleary eyed, exhausted, and begged him to hand me the baby. He threw my son at me and stormed out. As I lay there with my screaming seven-week-old, all I could think was: This can't be my life, this can't be my son's life, this isn't what I want for my child. This isn't the mom I wanted to be, broken and crying and scared. This isn't the relationship I wanted to model for my son. I called my parents to come get me. I packed up as much as I could with whatever energy I could muster between feeds. My husband thought I was just going with them to visit. As I sat down in the car, I felt the tension leave my body. A week later, I decided that I wanted a divorce and haven't looked back. My son gave me that strength—him growing up in a happy, stable home is all that matters. ***Being a single mom is hard, but my being a mom in a broken relationship was much harder.*** Now, both my son and I are happy and healthy, in every way. Mamas, just know that you are brave if you leave, and you are brave if you stay.

-Anonymous

S tarting a family with my first husband was so overwhelming because it was all on me. I went to this moms' group, and everyone was raging and angry about their husbands. One woman said, "Hired help is expensive, but divorce is more expensive." I never really had a lot of help from my first husband, but in retrospect, we should have hired some. I couldn't sleep because I was so angry all the time. My ex-husband needed more sleep because he worked twenty-four-hour shifts. Then, when he came home from work, or on his days off, I got nothing. I needed to hand off the baby for an hour, but my husband would come home and work out while I made dinner with the baby bouncing away in the carrier. He went out every Friday and Saturday, and then he would want to sleep in. And I was just like, I hate you. I don't even like you a little bit, I just actually hate you. ***No one tells you how hard a baby is on your relationship. Having a kid together fucks shit up, and nobody tells you that.*** This time I feel lucky. The difference with my new husband is that we genuinely appreciate each other's role. He takes the baby from 9 p.m. to 1 a.m., and I take him the rest of the night. And he is so grateful for what I do every day. If my ex ever said thank you, it was always with the tone of "thanks for doing your job." Now I have a partner in this, and it changes everything. It's not that it's not hard, because I still never sleep, but it's just so different. There are so many women going through what I did because they don't know anything different. Someone once said to me, "Being married is like having a sleepover with your best friend every night." It was the first time I realized that other people feel that way about their husbands and that I never would. The thought of getting a divorce was so scary. I thought and cried about it for a year and a half straight. I am so much happier now, and I am so glad and grateful. I wish that I could tell anyone going through it that it will be okay, and your kids will be okay. Everyone deserves to be happy.

-Anonymous

I met my ex-husband on a dating app when I was twenty-one. There were lots of good things about him: he was attractive, he was fun, he was charming. It all seemed great, but there started to be little things like him making comments about my weight, not liking body hair, or resenting how much time I spent with my friends. I viewed it as him caring about me and not so much as criticism. But the more time we spent together, the more critical he became, and there kept being a higher bar to keep him happy. Then we got engaged, and that's when things started to get really bad. We had a lot of fights and came close to calling off the wedding, but I was mortified at the idea. Little did I know I'd become a single mom of a three-week-old baby.

I got pregnant right away and had a miscarriage. The night of my miscarriage, he went to play soccer and have drinks and stay out with friends. I got pregnant again, and when I was twenty-seven weeks, I went to the bathroom and started pouring blood. I was admitted to the hospital and stayed there for a month. While I was there, he was very angry at me. He'd claim that no one was home to take care of him. He kept blaming me, saying it was my fault. It was very upsetting. His biggest concern at the hospital was what my parents would order him for dinner to eat that night. When they told me I could go home, I didn't want to.

I ended up back in the hospital with more bleeding, but I was happy to be there because I wasn't going home to him expecting me to do all this stuff for him when I was supposed to be on bed rest. I did not enjoy a moment of my pregnancy. The day I was going to get induced, my water broke, and I called him. He said, "I'm going to go to sleep and I will come when I get up in the morning." I was freaking out, as I didn't want to be alone.

My parents came, but he wasn't there until well into the induction process. He arrived as I was having contractions and he needed to write an out-of-office note. The nurse rolled her eyes at my mom as I had contractions while telling him what to write. Then our daughter was born.

She was four pounds, and as soon as she was born, he didn't think that anybody should hold her (this was pre-COVID-19). He sent me texts like, "Stop having our daughter passed around like a football." "What's wrong with you?" "What are you thinking?" "What kind of mother are you?"

I was having trouble breastfeeding, and he said, "I refuse to see my daughter have formula." He would remind me about what the lactation consultant said, which doesn't help when you're stressed. We stayed at the hospital for a week, but he slept at home because he needed his beauty sleep. When I got home, he didn't want my family or friends over; he didn't want anyone around. He also didn't want me to leave the house. I went against everything he said because I needed my family, and I needed to get out. There was one night when our daughter was two weeks old and I just wanted to grab a coffee with my friend and leave her with him for a half hour, and he said, "If she cries or is upset, I'm not letting you know. This is your fault for leaving."

I went out with my friend, I bawled my eyes out, and I told my friend that I couldn't do it. I didn't want my daughter to grow up thinking that this is how a woman should be treated. I spoke to my parents, and they were extremely supportive. At three weeks postpartum, I told him that I wanted a separation. He told his family I lost my mind and that I had postpartum psychosis.

Everybody in his family thought I had gone crazy. I hadn't gone crazy; it was the most sane and strongest I had ever felt.

When you separate with a newborn, there needs to be a parenting agreement before anyone can leave the marital home. I offered him a lot, but nothing was good enough, so I ended up being stuck in our home until she was four months old. One night I had had enough, and I pushed his buttons. It was stupid things that the average person wouldn't care about: things like eating his leftovers and using his expensive cream. I had been sleeping in the guest room, but that night I got back into the king-sized marital bed and said, "I'm sleeping here." That night, he forced himself on me and sexually assaulted me. I called my lawyer, who spoke to all the partners at the firm, and they told me to leave the house regardless of the parenting agreement—it was an issue of safety. My best friend and her husband came over, and I packed up my whole life in three hours. I took everything I could take, and that was it. I was gone.

We had four years of tumultuous legal battles, and we finally came to an agreement a year and a half ago. A few months after that, he got a job in another country. He comes back infrequently, and we actually get along fine now, which is shocking. It's taken a lot on my end: patience and forgiveness. ***My daughter is the best thing in the world, so I don't regret meeting him, but I know I deserve a lot more for myself, and hopefully one day I'll find it.***

—Anonymous

I *got the go-ahead to have sex after my six-week checkup. I don't know how long we waited after that, but every moment was painful.* My face was in the pillow, and I was crying. That went on literally for months. He was worried that he was hurting me, and I would say, "Just keep going, just finish, just keep going." That went on for a long time. No position was helpful at all. No joke, it still feels like something doesn't feel right. It took a long time, and it took a lot of taking one for the team to make it work. I would literally tell him to just do it so it would get better. It was like breaking my hymen again. It's just crazy because they tell you that even within that six-week phase you're in menopause, essentially, and you're completely dried up, which is the reason it hurt so much. You've got this new tight vagina like a teenager, except it's totally used and abused, so you have to have terrible sex, lose your hymen, and take one for the team, all at the same time.

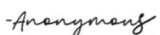

-Anonymous

W hen I first got pregnant, I wasn't concerned about my then-husband, but if I think about it now, being out of the marriage, there were terrible signs.

We found out the sex of the baby at the ultrasound (it was a girl), and that's supposed to be a very enjoyable and special time for expecting parents. But my ex yelled at me, screaming because he was so upset we were having a girl. I was in shock. You never think finding the sex of your baby would be like that.

After I gave birth, my daughter was tongue-tied, so breastfeeding was very painful. I'd cry in the middle of the night while breastfeeding, and he would stand over me screaming, "What's wrong with you? Everyone in the world can breastfeed and you can't, which means you're a horrible person."

I didn't talk to anyone about the abuse because I guess I normalized it. Most people didn't know what was going on until there was a breaking point and I had to start letting people in and explain what was going on. And I think about that a lot now. Thank God I got out before COVID. I know what it was like being stuck home with a child in an abusive relationship, and I don't know how people who are at home right now are dealing with it.

It took me a while to leave him. At first, I thought that I couldn't get divorced. I didn't know anyone who was divorced. *My biggest fear was that my child was going to grow up in a broken family.* Now I know she is so much better off with divorced parents than she would have been with us together, but it took a really long time to understand that. People say you have to stay together for the kids, but it's actually horrible for the kids to be in a relationship like that. It took two years and a lot of people—therapists, my family, and my friends—to get me to a point where I was strong enough to make that decision.

My motherhood experience after separating from my partner has been more positive because I wasn't my true self in the way I parented. I was in an abusive relationship, so I felt limited in what I could and couldn't do. I wasn't being the mother I know I'm capable of being. To be able to mother my daughter to the best of my ability now feels very powerful.

-Anonymous

Husbands and partners get a bad rap. Moms always talk shit about them. But it's so true. All of it. ***I didn't really have empathy for my husband because I felt so sorry for myself.*** He wasn't as naturally connected to the baby as I was. It makes sense. He didn't grow the baby, and once she came, he was limited in what he could do. He didn't know how to help her, and because she was exclusively breastfed, it was even harder for him. He couldn't feed her; he didn't feel comfortable bathing her; he didn't even feel that comfortable holding her, so it caused a lot of friction. I would jab at him about it, and he would get so sensitive. I felt bad because I knew if he could, he would. I wanted to help him and give him that confidence, so I spoke to a few friends who had older babies and asked how they did it. They allocated bath time or another routine to their husbands and made it their thing. My husband is wonderful, but he's a little awkward. I was so worried that he would drop her or something. I had to let go. I had to trust and empower him. Now he does bath time with her every day, and it's given them a time to bond. And I get ten minutes to myself. It hasn't stopped me from taking jabs at my husband, but it has helped us both manage our new reality.

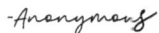

-Anonymous

We broke up four days ago. We did not make it. Relationships are not easy, and that's something a lot of people don't talk about. ***You need to be in a relationship and have a child with someone who wants the same things and is willing to make it work because it is like a job.*** It's exhausting to want to work on a relationship when the other person doesn't. We talked about going to counseling, but he was adamant about not going. If you can identify having certain issues, but you don't want to fix them, what does that say? For whatever reason, we're not important enough for him to do the work, which sucks because we were together for five years. We had problems within the first week of her being born. I was lying in a room with the baby trying to figure out breastfeeding. I still looked five months pregnant. He got up and made himself bacon and eggs. I could smell coffee brewing in the kitchen, and I thought he was actually going to bring me breakfast in bed. But he didn't even think about me. Tears were streaming down my face as I struggled to get her to latch, and I saw him walk by the bedroom and sit down in front of the TV to eat his breakfast. I was so mad that I thought my head was going to fly off my shoulders. I can't even take a fucking shit because I'm scared that my vag and asshole are going to rip open, and he's making bacon and eggs.

It took several months to work through my own feelings, to put my ego aside, and to understand what happened wasn't really about me—it was about him and where he was at. I've been a single mom for a year, and I'm comfortable in this new role, but I was embarrassed about it. And with all the BLM stuff happening, maybe my ethnicity was a factor because I didn't want to be a stereotype. Nobody really knew about what was going on. I kept it really private except for my inner circle. I was busier at work than I had been in a very long time. I was on set every other day, shooting commercials and memorizing lines. It felt like I was living in this parallel universe or was on a Ferris wheel that you just want to shut down—get me off this thing! And then when things finally calmed down, I was able to digest, think, and journal a lot. It was December 31, and my Instagram followers sensed there was some disruption in my life. I felt they should know why I was unraveling. I posted a ten-minute video on IGTV that mentioned the separation and my hopes and dreams for our next steps. In hindsight, speaking about how I envisioned our relationship 2.0 was probably manifesting it. I just wanted to leave all those negative, hard, hurtful, and emotional feelings in 2019 so they wouldn't carry into the new year! And then after the holidays, my nanny reminded me of an old Oprah line: "People can't meet you where you are, they can only meet you where they are at."

My daughter really wanted to go to the CN Tower in Toronto. I thought it would be a great activity for her dad to join us. I didn't want him to miss out on a first experience, whether he thought it was important or not. I just knew how I would feel if I wasn't included in a moment like that. So, I thought it was an opportunity for personal growth and a way for us to hopefully share a beautiful experience together with our daughter. I invited him, and as uncomfortable as it was, there was no arguing, there were no tears, and there was no frustration. Instead, there were a lot of smiles and laughs. It was tough in the sense that this was supposed to be our life. But that was outweighed by my daughter's squealing, giggling, and the elated look on her face. That moment changed the trajectory of our dynamic, friendship, and relationship. It was so positive that we now hang out a couple times a month as a family. Our daughter is the glue that keeps us together, and we both use her as a compass for anything that we do now. We just think about how it's going to affect her. My daughter had just turned two when we separated, so she couldn't process it. She's now starting to understand that our family dynamic is different from other families'. She was throwing fits and wanting her dad around at bath time and bedtime, which made me really sad. But now we are in a place where he can come over in the evening and help out. For her birthday, we celebrated at home because of COVID. He stayed after she went to sleep, and we just talked. We enjoyed hanging out, and it was hard, but I'd rather have that than a situation where we can't stand each other and need a third party to do the kid exchange. It's not perfect—we argue from time to time. I see how it impacts my daughter. She picks up on that energy, and she's just way happier when things are in an uplifting space.

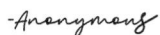

-Anonymous

***I* don't know if I could go through it again with my husband. I love him, but we've had this issue where I need him to step up when I can't, and he doesn't.** I don't get that choice. I have to put everything aside about how I'm feeling because someone needs to take care of this baby. Then I resent him, and he resents me for resenting him. It's hard. You change when you have a baby, especially in the fourth trimester. It's a huge thing that no one talks about. Your partner gets to shower every morning. They get to put on a new outfit. And they get to go about their everyday life. He sees his friends, and he gets to drink and have fun. And I'm at home with puke on me. I feel bad for him at times. We got into a huge fight recently where he said, "But it's hard on me too." I get it. I feel like I've tried to make our relationship equal for so long that I created a bit of a problem. It's not equal right now. I've just birthed a baby. I have all the hormones and feel like I've lost my career. So right now, it has to be just about me.

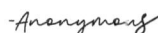
-Anonymous

No one tells you how hard it's going to be on your relationship. Because you take everything out on each other. Because you can't take it out on the kids. ***Parenting is sacrificing your "me" time and you do it for the kids, but there is this little folder in my brain that knows all the time my husband gets for himself.*** I file it. He is not a serious person. He jokes a lot, and it's kind of like his love language. It makes me insane. He came home yesterday and made a joke about how he has to go to work and make money while I get to be home. Must be nice and relaxing. He always makes those stupid jokes, and it makes me insane because it's so insensitive. This morning I sent him a text because yesterday he made another stupid comment about how nice it is to be at home. I said, "I know you think I do nothing all day, but since 9 a.m. (and this is at 11) I've gotten three people up and dressed, teeth brushed, I've fed two kids, dropped one off at daycare, cleaned the bathroom, taken out the garbage and recycling, stripped the beds, steam-cleaned the pee off the mattress, started laundry, called my dad, and got a baby to sleep." He wrote back, "Woah. By the way, I don't actually think you do nothing. Give me some credit."

-Anonymous

My husband knows me. We've been together long enough that he understands me. Recently, something he said, which was very kind but also so fucking annoying was, "How can I help?"

Don't fucking make me do that work for you. You figure out how to help and do it. I just feel like right now we are in the worst place. We're not speaking about splitting up, but we're definitely in a terrible place in our marriage. I just really dislike him, and he dislikes me, even though we love each other. There's just so much resentment. The sleep deprivation hits me the most, and it's what I'm most resentful about. ***Sometimes my husband wakes up after a full night sleep and jokes that the baby slept through the night, and I'm like go fuck yourself.*** People don't talk about how much you hate your spouse. For so long, I never understood divorce. Now I get it. I totally get it. At least we're on the same page in terms of not wanting to talk to each other. I met my husband when I was fifteen, and I often wonder if I would have pictured this—all this. I don't know.

-Anonymous

One of my biggest challenges is connecting with my husband. I am a very social person. I chat with everyone. I'm energized in social settings, and my husband is not. That was fine before kids because I had other outlets. With kids, there is so much more pressure on the relationship because I am home more and my husband has to fill the social void. We are constantly ebbing and flowing. We have great times where everything is going smoothly, and then it's like we haven't talked, gone for a meal, or even just sat down for dinner in weeks. That is the biggest challenge with a growing family. He has a full day of work, he runs his own business, and he's super stressed out all the time. It's hard for him. It's the same way I feel when giving to the kids all day long. I feel completely depleted and my glass is empty, and I am looking to him to fill it. Communication is the most important and hardest part. It doesn't come naturally to him. I am comfortable being vulnerable, talking and putting myself out there. We have never sought counseling, but we've had conversations where we have said that we need a third party to help us. We have three kids now, so do we have room in our lives for each other? We have to make room and time, but it's mostly working on being able to communicate. It's so hard. There has been an adjustment with each child. ***You are giving so much to a baby that you want someone to take care of you.*** It's a very hard thing for men to do, not just my husband. They have been taken care of their whole lives, starting with their moms, and then all of a sudden they have wives, and you have to walk him through it. If you don't talk about that stuff as a couple, you are doomed. We have been married for five years. We have had three kids in five years, and if we want one more, then our life is consumed by giving to our kids. If we fast-forward ten years from now and that's all we have been doing, then it's not going to work.

-Anonymous

I have no interest in sex at all. I don't see when that's going to happen. I feel bad because my husband is doing so much work to take care of us, and he wants to have sex but I don't. I haven't tried at all. I feel like I might be getting ready to try. Maybe? We've been sleeping with the baby in our bed, so if my husband comes near me to spoon, I say, "Get the fuck off me. Don't touch me." I don't even want him to go there. The past couple of weeks, I've been a bit better. I've let him cuddle me. It's baby steps. Eventually, I'll finally get there. But ***I just have no interest in sex. I've been holding a baby for every second of the entire day—I'm touched out.*** And the baby is on my nipple all day. So, boobs are off limits, don't touch my stomach—the sex is just going to be bad. It may as well just not happen. We also couldn't do it the whole time I was pregnant because I was on bed rest, so it's been a long time. I hope it's crazy when we do, but I feel like making time for it is something I'm going to have to consciously work on going forward. When you haven't had sex in so long, it's hard to jumpstart it. It's hard to even get into the mind frame for it. My mind frame is always the baby. It's just always in my head, and as you can imagine, babies are the antithesis of sexy.

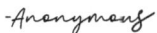
—Anonymous

When my water broke at 5 a.m. and we got to the hospital, my husband said, "I have a meeting tonight, so I really hope this isn't going to be a long labor." I got into the room, and he kept leaving. The midwife offered me comfort and held my hands and my feet during my contractions instead of my husband, because he kept dicking off. Then I was fully dilated, and my husband was still nowhere to be found. My midwife said it was time to push, so I called him three times. No answer. I left a message saying, "If you want to see your kid being born, you should come back," and he reappeared. I couldn't even get mad at him because there was no point. He is consistently like that. I gave birth at 11 a.m., and what did he say to me? "I can still make it to my meeting." My midwife said to me, "I can't let you leave the hospital if you are going to be home by yourself." So I lied, saying my whole family would be there. I wanted out of the hospital. She said I couldn't be alone with the baby because I just had an epidural and couldn't move my legs, but I lied. I said someone would be there with me. My husband brought me home, he brought me and the baby upstairs, then he took a shower and left. I was stewing in anger. ***The day after we had our baby, he went out, and it made me so jealous.*** Nothing changes for them. Their vagina isn't bleeding, boobs aren't engorged, they don't have excess skin, and they didn't get stretch marks. I got really bad stretch marks this time, and my husband really downplayed it, but if he gets one gray hair, I have to hear about it for a month. That part sucked. He just gets to go wherever he wants. It's really frustrating, and he makes me go from 0 to 100. I just can't handle it. I turn into the Hulk; I just go crazy. He always blames it on my hormones, and it's not that. He is just a dickwad. It's not hormones that make what he is doing wrong. It's not my hormones that justify that.

-Anonymous

In talking to so many women, we've heard about a great tactic for managing some of the most common conflicts that arise in relationships: make a list of the roles and responsibilities in the home and agree on who will do what and when.

Another way to clear the air in common relationship conflicts is to have a communication bible. It's a way to understand how to speak to each other during tense times.

Example: When I'm feeling frustrated, I need you to _____

Setting expectations as early as possible helps to really smooth the natural tension that can arise.

9

NO ONE EVER TOLD ME
HOW MUCH I'D NEED A VILLAGE.

You'll get by with a little help from your friends …

Mental health and depression.
If you feel like you might be experiencing signs of postpartum anxiety
or depression, we encourage you to consult a medical professional.

A s a new mom, things were difficult, but I still felt supported by my family and friends. I made sure I had stability and connection with other moms. I didn't even join social media until I had a baby, but I had to meet new people and make new friends. I was able to be a lot more honest about certain things. I was struggling with how to get through the really challenging early days of having a kid. That was super helpful, regardless of what was happening. I didn't focus a lot on self-care or self-reflection. I didn't do enough of that, in retrospect. I kept myself busy and wanted to distract myself by being social, but I also did get a lot from it. It did feed me a lot—making close friends with other moms. You find your women, you have your chat group, and then you're constantly connected. ***You can message someone at three in the morning for something and someone else is probably awake. Having that parallel experience with so many people is a huge way of getting through it.***

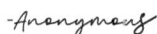

—Anonymous

I ***struggle socially to interact with other moms.*** In hindsight, I could have maybe tried to connect with other moms prenatally, but I didn't. I never really thought it would be so isolating. I've started to meet people by walking around. The stroller chat really works. I randomly met a girl while shopping, and we've become close. She comes to classes with me. There's another girl I've sort of become friends with, and we've gone on a few walks. You know the movie *I Love You, Man*? I feel like I'm Paul Rudd trying to find friends. I'm going on mom dates, and it's hard. I had a group my whole life, but I am the first one with a baby, so it's lonely. Some days the only person I talk to is the Starbucks barista until my husband comes home from work. And now that the days are really short and it's darker earlier, I feel like it's just going to be harder and harder. Some days it's rewarding and some days it's really hard. There are days when I sit upstairs in the nursing chair, rocking and crying. It's horrible, and you're alone, and you have no one because it's 3:30 in the afternoon. It always feels like you're the only person in the whole world who is there—and that's not the case. You feel alone, but everyone is going through it too. I didn't even think to do classes until a girl I know mentioned it. Now she is my social leader. I'm very grateful for her.

-Anonymous

P eople are in shock and awe when they learn I'm a mom of three kids under four. I'm often asked how I do it, but I don't know. We are barely doing it, and there's a perception that we have our shit together, but the reality is that we have a whole bunch of people in our village that make our lives function. I have a husband who does a lot around our home. Not just the bare minimum, but above and beyond what most parents would do. I had a nanny full time during the pandemic. My siblings and parents have also been supportive during COVID-19. The truth is that we have so many people in the background making things happen. ***I wish someone had told me sooner that building a community and having a village is not optional, it is mandatory.*** We need to combat the feelings of isolation and loneliness. We need to level up on our connections in motherhood because it is a lonely experience. We need to raise each other up. The pandemic has made us realize how much we need people until we don't have them. Friendship, girls' nights, walks, family, restaurants, concerts, travel—you never realize how important those moments are until you don't have them anymore.

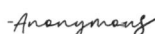
-Anonymous

B ecause I suffer from anxiety, I worried about developing postpartum anxiety (PPA) and postpartum depression (PPD) after giving birth. However, weeks and then months passed after my son was born, and I was seemingly okay. I experienced the regular hardships that new parents go through, intensified only by my newborn's colic and the witching hour that happened every evening like clockwork. *Once my baby turned five months old, I developed more and more feelings of anxiety and crippling depression that made me wonder if I loved my son as much as I should.* After consulting with my doctor, I was diagnosed with PPA and PPD. I wanted to be the best mom for my baby, so I immediately enrolled in group counseling at the local hospital. I attended the first class, then the following week the world went into lockdown because of COVID-19. I felt defeated but searched for online resources to help, and I found a virtual PPA/PPD counseling group that met once a week through Zoom. Each week I listened to fellow moms tell stories about their hardships, sharing tears through computer screens, and ultimately forming a bond that I didn't see coming. Once the classes ended, a couple of us decided to keep in touch via WhatsApp. And what I thought might be a supportive but short-lived chat turned into my biggest support system throughout my first year as a new mom. More than once, there were messages exchanged about our darkest inner feelings: like how we can be fit parents when we're carrying these demons? But then we would always reassure each other that we're in this together. The conversations have spanned hours and often turn from serious to lighthearted. We talk about everything from the latest treatment that we're pursuing for anxiety to the dreadful thought of sex post-baby. I've never met these women in person, but they know more about my deepest inner feelings than some of my best friends or closest family.

They're my village, and even though I'm still working through my PPA and PPD, I know that I'm not alone.

-Anonymous

***I*'ve become a vocal advocate of women and moms being able to have a safe space to talk about how they are really feeling, because I didn't have that.** I felt so alone and alienated. A close friend had a baby six months after I did, and we started a mom chat, just the two of us, where we would be super honest about how we were feeling. And the chat has grown to eight women. Every time a friend becomes a mom, we bring her into the chat, and it's a place where you can talk shit about your husband, talk shit about your kids, talk shit about how you're feeling, and no one is going to judge you. We are all here for each other. The other day one of the moms said, "I thank God every day for this space that you have created where we can talk. My best friend just had a baby who is colicky. One day she called me and said, 'I am so sorry for what I said to you when you were pregnant, now I understand.'"

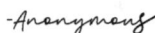
-Anonymous

You always think that everyone will help you when you have a baby, especially your family. My older sister was helpful, but she is super busy with three kids. My mom lives close by. She often comes over, but she will hold the baby and then be like, "Oh, can you just make me a bagel?" ***Anytime my mom offers to come over, I know that I'm going to have to take care of the baby and her.*** She never takes the baby and lets me do anything like shower. I was angry but should have expected it because my sister who has three kids warned me about how unhelpful she is. She is anti-helpful. I think our moms forget how hard it is because it's been so long since they had us. They think we are all crazy. My mom always laughs about sleep stuff, but when I was a baby, they just basically put me in my room and shut the door. There was no "sleep training" or anything like that. They just didn't care or didn't know. They didn't have video monitors or heartbeat monitors. What we do might be excessive, but it's a result of our generation having more knowledge available. People don't smoke in their houses anymore because we know more now. My mom used to put me in the crib with a bottle of apple juice. Who would ever do that now?

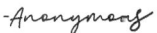

-Anonymous

I'm an introvert. I had to change for my kids. I'm not the most social person. I like doing my own thing. My friends are all older, and their kids are all older, so I decided I have to break out of my shell if my son's going to make friends. It's hard to let down your guard and try to make mom friends. What the hell! We're adults! Shouldn't everyone just be nice to everyone? But it's not like that. ***So many of us feel alone or like all these moms are judgy and unapproachable.*** We're all grownups now, aren't we? So why does it still feel a little like high school? It should just be civil and kind. We don't need to judge each other on anything. It's interesting. I've noticed it can be clique-like. You just have to kind of find your own village. You create your own village.

—Anonymous

I got really lucky with this group of girls because there is no judgment. On any given night at 2 a.m., we are all on WhatsApp talking to each other. It was something that I spearheaded. I did a prenatal class with a few girls, and we all had our babies over about two months. We did another class together, and more people joined this group. Now there are twelve of us. It goes on all day and all hours of the night. Any question we have. You can always just ask the group and they will have something. We all give advice. Right now on my phone, there are twenty-six messages, all from this group. If I put my phone down for two hours, I could have 150 messages. We do classes with each other all week. We do music, hangouts, and programs. These babies have been friends since birth, but really, it's for the moms. We also do a night out once a month. We all get together and do activities too. We did a really cute pumpkin patch day in the fall. We all say we don't know what we would do without each other, because it saves us. We know each other's babies so well. Literally, I could tell you their sleep schedules, poo schedules, what illnesses they've had—all of that. There is no drama in the group, and I think we achieved that because we refuse to judge. We are all going through this. Yes, there are some people who are really high strung, some who are really loosey-goosey, some who are super chill, and then some who are in the middle of the line. Is everybody going to be best friends? No. But we all still get along and have a really good balance in the group. When you're in those first few months together, everyone is just trying to figure it out, and you form a bond that is different from anything else. I think it's because we're all going through such a crazy time together and it's 2 a.m., and you're up talking. This group is so key to my enjoyment of being a new mom. There's so much I wouldn't have been able to do without their support. It's a resource you wouldn't even know existed.

-Anonymous

I am always on parenting forums. Facebook, Instagram—all the chats. They really do help. Man, what the hell did people do without their phones before? It's definitely a good and bad thing that we have so much access to information. With social media, you can definitely go into a spiral and start getting depressed if things aren't going well in your own life. ***Sometimes it can be really hard to see everyone's highlight reel. People only post their good stuff, so if you're struggling, that can be challenging.*** But I really do like the mom groups. Even if it's just a soap opera; even if it's just to entertain you for a few minutes. Just to watch all these people fight about breastfeeding or speculate about a rash. There's the drama of it all, but sometimes you get valuable information. I think it's probably a lot easier to be a mom now than it was pre-internet. People know more, and it's easier to connect with other people. There's still the older generation that thinks they know best. They grew up in such a different time that sometimes the advice they give is kind of hilarious. My mother-in-law recently told me to put the baby to bed on his stomach when we were having trouble settling him. She should get on Facebook and post that advice. That was quality drama.

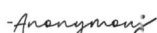
—Anonymous

I have so many good friends with young kids, not just with toddlers, but some with babies only a few weeks ahead of mine. So, there was almost a sense of betrayal in the sense that I didn't know what to expect. Like when I had my first panic attack. It was weird to find out that it is as common as first trimester nausea. I should have been expecting the panic attack, but I was so shocked with how alone I felt, especially when I spoke to all my friends and they said, "Oh yeah, I had mine at the pharmacy" or "My first one was when I was grocery shopping" or "My first one was the day my husband went back to work." It was so common that it should have been expected. So many emotions went through my head. Why didn't anyone tell me? I just felt so bad. I felt like a bad friend because I didn't know they were suffering so much. I felt like I needed to apologize to so many of my best friends because you can't understand it until you are going through it. Even if they did tell me that they were struggling and feeling down, I wouldn't have understood. I probably would have said the wrong things. ***I remember looking at my best friends and seeing in their eyes that they were suffering so much, but I didn't know how to offer that support or comfort or know what to do or say.*** There is so much suffering in silence. Why do we suffer in silence?

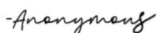
-Anonymous

Y*ou really need a partner. Well, you need a village, but that doesn't really happen anymore.*** I don't know how people do it alone. My parents are down the street, but they're not here for me emotionally. My parents would rather throw money at something than physically be here, which is fine—you take what you get. I would love the help though, especially having two kids. Picking up my son at daycare sucks. It's the worst time of day—it's the witching hour. It would be great to have someone be at my house so I didn't have to wake up the baby, put him in the car seat, and then have him scream the entire drive. I try to schedule it and strategize, but it's a little too far to walk and it gets dark so early, so I can't take the stroller. The double stroller won't even fit into the school. It would be nice to have that support but I don't have that from my family so much. You need a good partner for everything. My partner doesn't help with the baby so much this time around because he's so there for my older son. I need him to be. And let's be honest: if you're nursing, your partner can't do anything. It's not their fault. They don't have the milk. I feel bad because sometimes my husband will try to settle the baby and I tell him he's not doing it right. I have to remember that I'm here with the baby 24/7, and I'm learning every day. How can I expect him to just know? I took a postnatal class and the woman who ran it said, "Just walk away." Partners will figure it out and they need to learn too. This time around, he's there for my toddler. He gets him dressed in the morning, and he takes him to school. He doesn't complain, he just does it. It's what works for our family because now I'm finding it way harder to have a toddler than a baby.

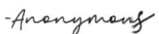

-Anonymous

One thing that no one tells you about is that other moms are bitches. Other moms are the worst people in the whole world. You would think we are there to build each other up, but that's not the case. I found a great group, but I have gotten so much judgment and criticism from other moms. They ask things like: "Are they doing this yet?" or "Why aren't you breastfeeding?" I was feeding my baby with a bottle in the park and this woman approached me and said, "That's what tits are for." I said, "You don't know me! How dare you say something like that!" She just walked away. People have no idea. I went to every lactation consultant, and they all said, "Keep doing it, keep doing it." But I didn't want too; I was just done. It was so hard and so stressful, and I wasn't able to just enjoy my baby. My best friend got really weird about bottle feeding too. She was constantly asking questions about our nursing experience or whether I was still trying. She told me to take fenugreek, and I just lost it. Why couldn't I just stop if breastfeeding wasn't working for me? But you can't. A mutual friend of ours finally had to tell her to stop. ***If breastfeeding works for you, that's amazing, but if it doesn't, you certainly don't need the added guilt and pressure from other women.*** We are supposed to be there for each other, not dragging each other down.

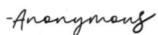

-Anonymous

Why is a village important to you? What do they do, or what do you wish they would do?

10

NO ONE EVER TOLD ME
HOW TO TAKE CARE OF MY MENTAL HEALTH AS A PARENT.

These stories contain references to postpartum depression and anxiety, as well as other mental health struggles faced by new parents. If you or anyone you know has concerns about your mental health, we encourage you to advocate for yourself and connect with a trusted healthcare provider.

Suicidal ideation, self harm, catastrophic thinking, and graphic content

T he baby blues hit me really quickly. A lot of the time I didn't understand why I was crying. ***Having the baby blues felt like someone turned on a faucet with my eyes.*** I kept wanting to relive that feeling of when my son was born and there was calm in the room. It was such a peaceful moment. Until last week, the baby blues were still really strong. The tears finally stopped, and hopefully it will stay that way. I have a history of depression, so it was a little scary for my husband. He would constantly ask, "Are you okay? Are you depressed? Do I need to be worried? Why are you crying?" I was super sensitive and super irritable. Luckily, my friend was checking on me every single day. My husband reached out to her. She said two to three weeks of baby blues is normal, but if it lasts longer than that it could be a red flag. People tell you about the baby blues, but I never understood what it was. Then I was wondering why I was crying so much. And you're tired, you're sore, you're getting lack of sleep, and you're not 100 percent down there. No one preps you for that at all. I have family members that are old school. They said, "You shouldn't cry, your milk can dry out." Everyone is telling you something different. My husband has been a lot of help. He stayed home with me for the first little while. I imagine the single moms who don't have any family or help. I praise them because this is not easy. They are superhumans.

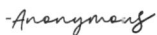

-Anonymous

The sleep deprivation caught up to me, and as time went on, my anxiety was getting worse. When I weaned my daughter, my anxiety kicked into high gear. I know there is a big shift in hormones, but it quickly turned into depression. It was not one of those situations where I was stuck inside and isolated. I had a decent social life, and I was working part time. It just kicked in. It goes to show that no one is really immune to postpartum depression. You could be fine, and then all of a sudden you're not. I was learning to manage this new life with two kids who have very different needs while trying not to feel like a failure. I started to think that my family might be better off without me. That I was not doing a good enough job as a mother. That my husband didn't find me attractive anymore. Everything compounded. I remember driving home one day and thinking about how I would drive down to the lake and walk into the water and never come out. I am not a strong swimmer, so that would be the plan if I ever wanted to do that. I sat in my car and texted my friend: "Things are not good; I'm not well; I am having really dark thoughts and I need you to know." This is somebody I trust with my life, and she is the only person I told. I knew that by telling her, she would take it upon herself to check in on me and my kids to see how we were doing. I texted another friend who runs a mental health practice, and she connected me with a psychotherapist. I got an appointment the next week, and I started going weekly. Eventually, I told my friends and my husband. He didn't see it coming, and he wanted to know how it got so bad. I've been with him for sixteen years. He knows me really well, yet he didn't see postpartum depression kicking in. It's very silent. ***Postpartum depression is like being a prisoner in your own mind.*** You know that you have people around who love and need you, and you want to be there for them. But you're stuck in this cage in your mind being convinced they are going to be somehow better off without you. It's a really weird place to be.

-Anonymous

I was thirty-four when I had my son and most of my friends were on their second or third kid already, so I felt like I had tried to plan everything that I could to prepare myself for how hard it would be, especially the fourth trimester.

Before the haze of the fourth trimester wore off, the pandemic hit. There was so much uncertainty that I think it really triggered something in my brain.

I've done a lot of therapy. I do individual therapy and group therapy, and I've been trying to figure out when it got really bad, but I see it as an accumulation of things, and I think that's what happens to a lot of people.

I think the first thing that started the train in motion was when my son was two days old and we had to go to a breastfeeding clinic. I had a breast reduction when I was eighteen and was having some issues feeding. We were referred to this clinic, and I thought we were going to talk about getting breastfeeding under control. He had dropped a lot of weight, and no one had ever talked to me about how common that is. The lactation consultant and the doctor came in and sat us down. It just felt so serious. They said, "Listen, we are going to have to talk about formula." Right away, I felt like a failure. I assumed we would figure it out, but it was the first time I felt the magnitude of it, this life-or-death thing that started becoming very prevalent throughout my whole postpartum journey. I assumed that breastfeeding would hurt and be stressful, but I didn't realize it would feel like if you don't feed your baby enough, he could die.

It started with that, and then a week later, I started breaking out in postpartum hives. It was unbearable, and it's something that people don't talk about but is common. I saw an allergist, and she said a lot of women postpartum do have an autoimmune response to not being pregnant anymore and so your body just freaks out. I had these hives, I was so uncomfortable, and I was pumping around the clock, breastfeeding and not sleeping.

Because of the pandemic, I pushed through breastfeeding. The state of my breasts at that time was disgusting. I would pump blood, but I kept going because I had read in the news that the antibodies in breastmilk may help your baby. There was this constant narrative to me that everything was life or death. I had to do these things to keep my baby alive. I had it in my head that he needed the nutrients from breastfeeding for his immune system or he would die. We didn't know much about COVID and babies then, so it was playing into that fear.

Then I started having visions all day long of my son dying. He was learning how to crawl and was eating solids, which are two big milestones, but every time he did something, I could see how he could die. If he stood at the doors, I would picture him falling and cracking his head open. If he would gag, I would see him choking. It was a constant narrative of death. I started having panic attacks.

My husband had no idea that any of this was going on, but on one occasion I mentioned something to him, and he was shocked. It was the first time I thought that this might not be normal. There were a few other instances when I had panic attacks and these really overwhelming thoughts, but they weren't like in the movies. In the movies, people zone out and they have this flash, and then they come out of it. For me, it was just this quick vision in the back of my mind, but ***because it wasn't like I'd seen it on TV, I hadn't thought it was a sign of postpartum depression or mental health issues.***

One of the only times I saw my family during the pandemic, I had a panic attack around them, and my sister said that I needed to get help. So, I started therapy, and it's helped a lot. Just with processing my thoughts and knowing that it's not real. Yes, something bad could happen, but it probably won't. I'm not 100 percent yet, but it's helping to take some of the weight off. And I feel like the pandemic made it so hard because if I had been around people, maybe someone would have seen it and I could have gotten help earlier.

-Anonymous

I hear many moms say they dreamed of becoming a mother. I definitely did not. I don't look back fondly on my childhood. My parents were dominant, and my mother suffered from untreated depression. It was always like walking on eggshells trying not to set them off for my own emotional and physical safety. I had this fear that if I became a parent, it would become a generational pattern and I would repeat the same behavior. I had heard so many times that you do what you know. Fast-forward to when I was thirty-two. I struggled in relationships until I met this compassionate, understanding, and loving man who became my husband. We talked about having kids, and I was honest about my fears. I also thought my likelihood of getting pregnant was low because I have Polycystic ovary syndrome (PCOS) and I had thyroid cancer. I felt it was the universe's way of ensuring I didn't have kids. My husband reassured me that I could be a good mom regardless of the way I was parented. He gave the example of how much I cared for my dog. But I said that it was a dog, not a human, so totally different. He said it still showed I could be nurturing and loving. He also assured me I would have the support of his family. I had no family in the city, so I was scared not to have a village and to feel suffocated by motherhood. We made the decision to try to get pregnant with no expectations. We had just moved into a new home, and two months later, I was pregnant. I was scared shitless. I started reading books on attachment parenting because I wanted to raise my child in the complete opposite way I had been raised. I wanted a natural birth, an unmedicated labor, and to breastfeed my baby exclusively. I was already a control freak, and I wanted everything to be just perfect. It turns out, there was so much I couldn't control.

As soon as my baby was born, it felt like things were spiraling downward. I struggled with nursing. I had not given it any thought while I was pregnant. I assumed it would come naturally. It was so hard. Giving up on nursing would feel like failing, and I didn't want to fail, no matter the cost to my emotional state. I wasn't breastfed, and I wanted to give my child all the things I didn't have. Gradually, nursing started to feel better, but I didn't. My son was still crying a lot. The witching hour went on for several hours. I would be home crying, pacing, and anxiously waiting for my husband to come home from work to take him off my hands. I would go to my room, shut the door, and cry some more. I had all this resentment from feeling like I was alone. Where was the support my husband and his family had promised me? This was my worst nightmare coming to life. I kept reading all these parenting books. I had always done well in school, so wasn't this the same thing? The visual I have of my journey into motherhood is swimming through mud. It was messy, and I didn't have confidence or a belief in myself. I was ashamed that I couldn't be the mother I saw outside my window. Everyone else seemed like they had it together. I isolated myself because no one was talking about how hard it was, so how could I? That first year took an emotional toll on me and my relationship with my husband. I blamed him for a lot of how I felt instead of accepting that I had a lot of work to do on healing myself. After my one-year mat leave, I went back to work. We had a nanny to help, and I felt like I could finally breathe again. But my son was extremely sensitive, and he would have big meltdowns, which were still triggering for me. I now feel a lot of his behaviors were mirroring how I was feeling. I still wasn't finding joy in motherhood. I didn't have the child I dreamed of. I hated myself for feeling that way. I wanted another child so that if I decided to walk away, they would at least have each other. How awful is that? Maybe I also secretly felt like it was my "take two." If I didn't have the dream experience with my first child, maybe I could have it with my second. But I realized I couldn't be the parent I wanted to be because I hadn't healed my inner child. All those triggers and limiting beliefs were still there. I hadn't made peace with the way I was parented. No book was going to do that for me. I had to confront my childhood trauma.

I am finally on a journey of healing. ***I truly believe that when you heal the mother, you heal the child.*** I also want to help other mothers heal themselves and be the best person and mother they can be. It has led me to begin a certification in peaceful parenting. I would never have thought this would be my life's purpose, but it feels like it has all come full circle. I am choosing to break the generational parenting pattern. It has taken eight years, and it will be a lifelong journey, but I finally feel I have stepped into my true self. I have a more connected relationship with my kids and my husband. I am learning to let go of the things I cannot control. I can be the person and parent I want to be.

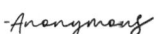
-Anonymous

We got pregnant during our investigative cycle at the fertility clinic. Everyone was so excited for us because we previously had had three miscarriages. There is a video of my dad holding up our daughter after she was born and it's like that moment in *The Lion King*. She had arrived. As I started to wean her off breastfeeding, I got pregnant again. I had my period the whole time, so I knew I was technically fertile, but since we had so much trouble getting pregnant the first time, it never crossed my mind that I could get pregnant accidentally. I didn't know I was pregnant for two months. And we were about to move. I was packed and about to leave everyone we love. And then I found out I was pregnant. I fucking lost my shit. I don't know if it was the hormonal change from not breastfeeding anymore, but I became so depressed. I had not recovered from just having my baby (she was just over five months when I got pregnant). So, when I found out, I was like, no, no, no, there's no way I'm keeping this child. I'm getting an abortion. I couldn't even stomach telling people I was pregnant. What were they going to think of me? I was going back to work, and we had just bought a house. I went into a really dark place and kept fantasizing about walking in front of a car: not to die, but to be injured enough to get hospitalized and have someone take care of me and I wouldn't have to be a mom for a while. Whenever someone would say congratulations, I would start crying because I was not in a place where I could hear it. ***I felt this guilt that my daughter would not have enough time as the only child.*** It got to the point where I didn't want to see anybody, and I didn't want to talk about my pregnancy. I didn't take any pictures because I didn't want to acknowledge that I was getting bigger. I finally realized that I had to take action and get help. I found a therapist who has been one of the greatest gifts of my life. It was such a safe space to meet, and she really helped me through the pregnancy and my thoughts and feelings. She helped me see it in a positive light. I had all this guilt and feelings of failure, and then my daughter was born and she was an angel baby. She was quiet, calm, sweet, and cuddly. I just fell so in love with her. It made my heart expand. I look at her every day and I think how less bright the world would be if I had had an abortion. She is the most amazing thing that could happen to us.

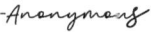

-Anonymous

Nobody talked to me about pregnancy, postpartum depression, and anxiety. I had the baby blues for three weeks. I thought I was in the clear, but things just weren't right, and I didn't realize that for about two years. At that point, I started to hear about postpartum anxiety for the first time—no medical professional had ever mentioned it to me. I had a lot of mom friends, but no one talks about how you're really, truly feeling on the inside. The word "anxiety" is thrown around so much, and I thought I was above that. But the more I started learning about postpartum anxiety, the more I thought I might have it. I'm the oldest of six siblings, and I work in childcare, so I was so sure I could be a mom. I'm a bit of a perfectionist. I got it in my head that I had to be a perfect mom, and I know it sounds cocky, but I was. I used all my energy and power to do all the right things, but I didn't realize how much I was depleted in every other aspect of my life. I didn't do anything for myself. I had no hobbies, my friendships started to diminish, and my marriage was shit. Then I got pregnant again. Adjusting to two kids is just a nightmare, and things started to diminish quickly. There were a lot of tears, a lot of adjustments, and a lot of fighting with my partner. I called my doctor when my son was eight months old because I knew something was wrong. I kept saying, "I'm not okay." My doctor asked if I could describe what was going on, and I explained that I was having really intrusive thoughts.

My thoughts were pretty graphic. For example, when I'd pass a car on the highway, I instantly envisioned a car accident and every detail after that. And I saw it a hundred different ways. I saw myself lying bloody, trying to crawl into the backseat. I'd try to get the baby out, and he's not breathing, or I'd see my daughter covered in blood and me trying to get her out. I had those kinds of thoughts constantly. I just thought they were normal mom worries, but I started to notice that they were taking over. ***I couldn't leave the house without thinking something catastrophic.*** My doctor recommended anxiety meds, but it felt too much like 0 to 100 for me. I wanted to try and come to terms with my anxiety and do what I could on my own. I started with a nutritionist because my physical health was so depleted. I'd focus so much on the kids and then it would be noon and I hadn't had any water. And then I'd be eating just their leftovers for dinner. I went to see a psychologist, and she diagnosed me with general anxiety disorder and postpartum anxiety. It was a huge sense of relief. Something was wrong with me, but now I could put a plan in place to get better. I cried for weeks after, not because I had anxiety, but because I had suffered alone for four years. I have so much regret. I wouldn't be in such a bad place if I got help back then. If someone had just said that I didn't seem okay, or if I knew that my thoughts were not okay, I could have done something sooner. I thought moms were just like that. Since being diagnosed, I have started to share my story so that other moms can think about their own health and consider whether they are okay or not.

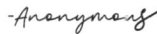
-Anonymous

I *had postpartum depression, and I am still managing it with therapy.* There is a cultural aspect to it. With South Asian culture, I was seen as the mother, this is just how it is, and we don't talk about these things because mental health isn't a real issue. You have to suck it up and not tell people about your vagina and not tell people you are depressed because the community is going to think you are crazy. It's a very old-world way of thinking about it. My family is quite different, but as liberal as they are and as open as I've been, they don't ever talk or ask about it. It's kind of disappointing because my postpartum anxiety is not just about me having the baby blues. This is me having thoughts of taking my own life. I don't know the extent of what my parents know, but I put everything out there on social media. And I know other family members have read things, but they don't ever ask about it. I really feel for parents who are in it for the first time and don't have a community to have these candid conversations. I have a history of depression, and I know it's really hard for people to ask for help. That's why I think it is so important for us to have a village, and it doesn't have to be our family, it can be our neighbors.

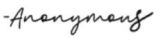

-Anonymous

When I got home from the hospital, there were a lot of people at my house, but I needed to sleep, so I went upstairs. When I got up, the trauma of what happened hit me like a ton of bricks. I was shaking uncontrollably, and my face was white. I called Telehealth and they told me to go to the walk-in clinic. The clinic sent me to the hospital because they thought I might have an infection. At the hospital, I found out I was having an anxiety attack, which turned into a full mental breakdown. I was obsessing over whether I had a fever, and I was taking my temperature every half hour. I was obsessing over my bowel movements. I made my doctor do a million tests. I made her do an ultrasound to make sure there was no residual blood stuck inside my uterus that could cause a postpartum hemorrhage. I did more blood tests because my fingers felt tingly. The problem with anxiety is that it makes you feel like it's all real. I thought my body was trying to tell me something. I felt like I needed to pay attention to it. And if I didn't and something happened, I would die. I was terrified that I was going to die. It's still there. It's a daily struggle for me. ***But everyone is dealing with something, and no one is talking about it. We have to be a team. We have to be able to talk to each other.***

-Anonymous

My son was born early, and he was very unhappy to be here. He would scream so loud that every night my husband would say, "We need to take this kid to a hospital." We'd never heard anything like it. His digestive tract just took time to work well, so he cried like that every single night for probably a month and a half. It was about two months in, and if you can describe rage in a color, it was white with no noise. I just completely lost it. ***I've never lost it like that in my life, but I was just going on one to two hours of sleep, and it was unbearable.*** I can't even remember what set me off. I just couldn't take it anymore. I went into the basement, and I punched the wall. Then I was lying in the laundry room and screaming. My husband was holding me, and I was pounding down on the concrete in the fetal position saying, "I can't do this anymore." It was one of those moments where you look back and it is complete madness, like you've completely lost control. I've never been that angry or upset or sleep deprived. It's an out-of-body experience. It's like you're a ghost—you're not you. Then I felt okay. I look back at that moment; my husband said he had never seen me that upset (and we've been together for thirteen years). I tend to get upset in a physical way sometimes. Not toward other people, but I've been known to punch a pillow to get it out. But this time I just had to run off. I ran to the basement and punched the wall and a picture fell off and hit the ground and broke. I was done. I just had nothing left in me anymore.

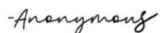

-Anonymous

I suffered from postpartum depression after my second. It was dark and miserable, and I didn't understand how I could divide myself between two kids under the age of two. It was the textbook situation that you hear about. but I had no one to talk to. My girlfriends hadn't gone through it, my sister-in-law hadn't gone through it, and my sister was busy dealing with twins. I felt like I was dealing with it alone. I sought professional help and, in doing so, geared up for the idea of having a third kid, which was really daunting. I carried a lot of guilt about how I was with the second: not feeling present in the first four months of his life and not feeling connected to him. It took more than 100 days to finally feel okay and feel like I had my shit together again. The third baby has been a completely different experience than my second. I don't think I suffered from anything this time. I knew the signs, symptoms, and what I needed to be a better mom and person. I asked for help when I felt like I needed it. I took time for myself when I felt like I was boiling over. I got people to help me, whether it was a night nurse, a nanny, or parents. ***I didn't pretend to be a hero, because in appearing to be a hero to everyone on the outside, I was suffering so deeply on my own.*** And now what you see is true. I am so happy, and the baby is thriving in a calm environment. It took three times to figure out my recipe for success as a mom, as a woman, and as someone who is still working and wants to find time for myself. We think we can do it on our own because we're moms and that's our role. And we think that having help is weak because we can't show weakness. Asking for help is not a form of weakness. Yes, you can do it on your own, but can you do it happier and better with help. There's something beautiful about our children being cared for by multiple people in different ways. You're not a bad mom if you take an hour to go to the gym or lie down while someone takes your baby for a walk. It's all part of the mental health journey that is such an enormous part of those 100 days.

-Anonymous

I truly believe postpartum blues isn't a joke. I loved my son immediately when I saw him. He was the tiniest little human I've met. Like a little man on a mission. He was born at thirty-five weeks, and although he was supposed to stay at the NICU, he defied all odds and avoided a stay. He passed all the requirements to be by my bedside. My first baby was delivered via C-section. This one was a vaginal birth, which I was so terrified about, especially when I developed a fever during labor. But he came out so fast, there was no time to do a Cesarean. I realized after that experience that whether a woman delivers via C-section or naturally, she will still be left with so much pain and soreness. I couldn't compare which was worse . . . my C-section recovery from my first pregnancy or my episiotomy pain and third-degree tear from this one. I hated what was happening down there. ***The feeling of love and the glow you're supposed to have turned into despair.*** I hated the after-birth pain so much. It was the most unglamourous feeling. How was I supposed to take care of two kids while not being able to move, sit, pee, or poo? Three days after birth, when my baby got the green light to come home, reality hit me. I was so overwhelmed with fear, sadness (no idea why), and the feeling that I would suck at being a mom of two. I cried in front of my husband at dinner time. While he reassured me that we would be okay and we would form a new routine soon and get used to our new normal, it was my toddler who somehow managed to squash my blues. He asked when he saw me crying at the table, "Mama, are you okay?" His sweet, innocent, two-year-old face made me nod in the middle of tears and forced a smile. "Yes, bubba. Mama is okay. We'll be okay." He thoughtfully considered what I said, then asked, "Do you want a Peppa Pig Band-Aid, Mama?" My sweet, sweet child.

I wish all worries and troubles could be fixed with a Peppa Pig Band-Aid. Knowing I have my family by my side, especially a toddler who showed empathy, love, and strength when I needed it the most, I decided right then and there NOT to allow the blues to take over my life as a new mom of two.

-Anonymous

11

NO ONE EVER TOLD ME
THAT MY STORY MIGHT NOT BE
WHAT I EXPECTED.

A section of stories from mothers who gave birth to
babies with health complications.

*The following two sections deal with babies born with health complications and
loss and grief. We realize that these stories can be difficult to read and may be
extremely triggering, but they are important and need to be told and heard. There
are no journal prompts in these sections, but we have included blank space at
the end in case you can relate and want to share your story. From experience,
getting heavy things off your chest doesn't change the circumstance, but it takes
the weight off, even if only a little bit. Your experience matters, and even if it's
not reflected in the following stories, you are not alone.*

I had preemie triplets, and when they were born, they looked normal. They made eye contact and they were smiley—all those kinds of things were fine. They were not meeting their milestones, but the doctors said it was because they were so premature. When you hear that milestones will be delayed for sure because they were premature, you don't really think that the worst could happen. I was so positive and naive in a way. I was trying to be positive, and I was positive for everyone around me. My parents were nervous, and I said, "It's going to be okay; they are going to be amazing, and I'm going to do everything for them," because I thought that I could control the situation. And then you can't. ***It was a blow like you can't even imagine when they were diagnosed with CP, because they give you this picture—it's a scale where they have the least severe to the most severe—and they showed me where my kids were on this scale, which was closer to the severe side.*** They showed me a cartoon of a child in a wheelchair with his head down, and it's impossible to imagine. I had a baby in my arms. They were babies, and to imagine that's what it will be and to project that on them was terrible. The doctors have experience with this. They've seen it a million times, but this was my first time seeing it, so it was not handled well. They are so desensitized to it, but it's like being punched in the stomach. Who are you to say that's going to be my kid? I'm going to do everything to make sure it's not.

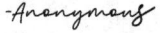

-Anonymous

I passed all the ultrasound and bloodwork tests when I was pregnant. But when my daughter was born, there were fifteen doctors in the room. They took her away, and I knew something was wrong. We found out she has Down syndrome. We didn't know what that meant. I was twenty-three and her dad was twenty. I questioned God and wondered why this happened to me. I am a good person, I go to church every weekend, I donate blood, I always try my best to help out . . . and then I find out I have a child with special needs. I noticed she was different as soon as she was born. Her body was really floppy. It wouldn't stay bent, and her legs were like frog legs. I had to carry her everywhere. I had a lot of help from therapists. They said I would have to do a lot of extra things for her and that it's not going to be an ordinary life. I was doing physical, developmental, and educational therapy. I took sign language classes because her speech would be delayed. It was hard to manage my time. When you have a child with special needs, you are so scared to put her into the hands of other people. I get so nervous leaving her with her grandma, but I need time for grocery shopping or just to have a little time to breathe.

Telling my family was hard. They thought it was a disease that one of us was carrying, and we had to explain the whole process of Down syndrome. In high school, they don't really explain any of that. They give you a toy doll in parenting class. You feed her, change her, and if you don't, you lose marks, but that's it. They don't cover a lot in those classes. I never took it seriously. So, when I had my daughter, it was a lot to take in. ***The world doesn't really accept a baby with a disability.*** It was hard being a first-time mom and dealing with the emotional stress. Right after I gave birth, one of the nurses scared me to death. She said, "Those babies are hard to take care of and some people put them up for adoption. You're a young mom; you're not ready for this job." I was so livid. I got that nurse's name, and I wrote a letter to the hospital. We were still processing her diagnosis, and it was not appropriate for her to say that. But that's common when you have a child with Down syndrome—you get that negativity. I am a young mom and the only one in my friend group with a child who is special needs. I took a completely different path than my friends. I lost a few friends, some cousins, and my older brother. I'm not close with him anymore because he is not supportive of Down syndrome. He just thinks I ruined my life. It's the hardest when it's family because you expect them to support you. But everyone is entitled to their own opinion. It's been hard, but I made new friends from the Down Syndrome Association group. I'm the youngest mom there.

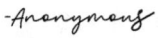

-Anonymous

I have a son. He is my only child, and he is awesome. He emulates a lot of his dad's personality: he's fearless, a go-getter, and happy. That's been a very big blessing because he wasn't brought into life in the most opportune way. During an anatomy scan while I was pregnant, the technician said, "Oh, I need to check something, I'll be right back." My gut was telling me something was wrong, and as the minutes passed by, I got more worried. It felt like forever, but she came back with the radiologist, and he told me they thought something was wrong with my baby's heart. It's so scary when you hear something about the heart. I went to a pediatric hospital and found out the baby had something called Tetralogy of Fallot, which is a congenital heart defect. Tetra is four, and it meant there were four issues with the heart. It's the same heart defect that Olympic snowboarder Shaun White has. Jimmy Kimmel's son has it as well. I had a choice of whether to go forward with the pregnancy or to terminate. They told me that kids with this condition need to have, at minimum, open-heart surgery, but often it requires immediate surgery when they are born—sort of like a Band-Aid surgery to get them to the big surgery. I was also told that sometimes these kids are born with a chromosomal deletion, which could mean they have Down syndrome or DiGeorge syndrome. To be honest, when they told me, my thought was that we would terminate the pregnancy. I didn't want to bring a kid into this world if they wouldn't have a good life. I could get an amnio that would tell us if the baby would have the chromosomal deletion. We decided that if the baby had the physical condition and deletion, we would terminate the pregnancy, but if it was just the heart condition, we would move forward. We had to wait ten days to get the results. The test came back negative, and we moved forward with the pregnancy.

My delivery was extremely planned out, and I knew the first hour of his life was going to be critical because they were looking at his oxygen saturation levels. Most people are around 100 percent, and there was a threshold where if his levels were below 80 percent, he would need immediate surgery as a precursor surgery to open-heart surgery. I delivered and I held him for ten seconds before they took him away to monitor. I had to wait three hours to see him again. We were fortunate that his heart condition was as favorable as possible. He didn't need surgery right away. They told me to treat him like a normal kid without limitations, and we tried to listen to that. I joined all these mom groups, but leading up to his surgery, I felt myself pulling away from them. I couldn't handle some of the questions they would post. They were things that first-time moms think about like what blanket should I use? But their concerns were so different from the things I was worried about at that time, so I felt like I had to pull away.

For his surgery, he had to be 100 percent healthy and we had to be 100 percent healthy, and that meant even a cold was an issue. They didn't tell us to go into social isolation, but we basically did because a lot of my friends' kids had hand-foot-and-mouth disease. We went on social lockdown for a whole month. It was the best thing for our physical health but the worst for my mental health. It was a hard time. I learned that there is a lack of mental health support for parents or expecting parents because they didn't really do anything for me at that point. I would have appreciated being recommended for counseling because it was fucking hard. They should have thought about and put more emphasis on proactive parental mental health. Even if you feel like you're coping, you need to advocate for yourself. That needs to be a big focus. Not just the well-being of your baby. If you're not okay, your baby won't be okay, and your family won't be okay. Every new parent goes through a lot of shit, and it's important to know that some kids don't come into this world healthy and the toll that has on becoming a new parent.

I'm a type A person, and it was hard. I had all these grand plans of what it would be like when he was born, and a big lesson I learned is that you can't plan anything. You need to make the best decisions that you can with what you know, but at the end of the day, you have to surrender.

-Anonymous

*I**n the last couple of years, there has been so much support and conversation around motherhood, but none of it has applied to my experience with a special needs child.*** You have to fit a very specific mold in order to access support, and when you don't—and most of us don't—you're truly left on your own. It started at my daughter's three-month appointment. We were meeting absolutely no milestones. The actual diagnosis came within the first year. She was born with zero muscle tone, which has affected everything: cognitive, physical, speech. Everything is slow and delayed. When she was in a special needs facility, I would often chat with some of the other moms, but it's very difficult to hear everyone else's shit storm when you're trying to keep afloat in your own. I felt like saying, "Woah, I can't get into this with you because it's dark and hard." Listening to other people's hell is not supportive for me. I have latched onto one or two people for help who are one step removed and talk to me objectively. One is a family member who is a speech therapist that works with special needs children. The other is a friend whose son went through a lot of challenges. But en masse, within the motherhood community, I've found that support is not there. There's a difference between asking for sleep training advice or tips versus something that you know no one can fix.

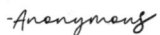

-Anonymous

I was never someone who dreamed of having children. My husband was more into having kids right away. I wanted more time, but he dreamed of having kids his entire life. I was never the most maternal person, and I was always worried that I wouldn't connect with my baby. When my son was born, they put him on me, and I know it sounds corny, but it does change you. Before it got too blissful, I looked up at my husband and he was totally white. He asked, "What's wrong with his ears?" The delivery doctor also turned white and said, "Oh, my God." What did they mean? They weren't telling me anything. They took the baby off me after two seconds so I didn't even have time to digest that he might not be healthy. A pediatrician came back with the baby and pulled my husband aside. They came back a few minutes later and the doctor started rambling. He said that my son was born without ears, and they don't know if he can hear. I was minutes post-labor, and I didn't understand what he was saying—it was so inappropriate. Thankfully, my delivery doctor said, "You can't speak to her this way; you need to walk away and we'll talk in a bit." We went to the post-op room and I wondered whether ears could grow. Can he hear? A new pediatrician came in and said, "I'm not sure what your son has, so take the night and we'll speak about this tomorrow." What did they mean, take the night?

We were eventually told that he has a condition called microtia. It's ten in a million. Aside from his ears, the doctor wasn't sure how the condition would impact my son, but we learned there was a possibility of kidney and heart failure. I had just gotten over the fact that my kid might not be able to hear, and then they dropped that on me. They gave him an ultrasound on his kidneys, and while we were in the ultrasound room, they slammed the door. The nurse said, "I think he heard that." Then we started wondering if he could hear. Those were my first twenty-four hours as a mom. and I was drowning—beyond drowning.

They released us, and within the first two weeks, we checked his ears, kidneys, and heart. I flew to Chicago to get a developmental assessment. We discovered that his inner ear works, but not the outer ear. He can hear perfectly, but the sound can't come in because it's blocked. The good news is his speech and language will develop perfectly normal without impediments. He's only a little bit delayed because he couldn't hear in utero, but he will catch up. So, I wanted to give him the opportunity to hear as soon as possible. You are their only advocate. ***If you are not your child's advocate, you will fall through the cracks very quickly.*** Putting on the hearing aid was amazing. I didn't know if he would react because he was three weeks old, but he just became so much more alert. He's the most social baby. I know it sounds corny, but I think he was born to us for a reason. When I said I wasn't a maternal person, it changed the second they put him on me and I was told something was wrong. I felt the instinct right away at that moment. I needed to protect him. You drop everything. Nothing else matters other than giving your kid the best life and opportunities. They offered to put the hearing aid in the back of his head to be more discreet, but I knew it was better in the front. If he can hear better with it on the top of his head, then that's where he is going to wear it. He wears a headband to support the hearing aid. When my mom got married, the photographer asked if I wanted to remove the headband, and I said no. I want him to look back on photos and know who he was. I never want him to feel like I'm embarrassed of him or that I care that he has microtia. During the first six months, I cried every night. I never wanted him to feel any of my stress or anxiety so any time I got upset, I went upstairs for a few minutes. I want him to feel like it isn't a big deal because in the grand scheme of things, it isn't. I'm hopeful that he's not going to have the hearing aid forever, but even if he does, he's going to be able to hear his whole life.

-Anonymous

12

NO ONE EVER TOLD ME
THAT I'M NOT THE ONLY ONE.

This section is devoted to those heavy topics like
miscarriage and loss. If you have recently gone
through loss, we recommend that you skip this section until you feel ready.

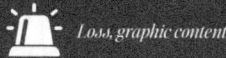 *Loss, graphic content.*

I*t's crazy how in the span of twenty-four hours, you can go from anticipating the best day of your life to experiencing the worst.* Life can change in an instant, and unfortunately, we don't realize how important cherishing every moment and living life to the fullest is until that change happens. It's a reminder to hold back from looking at our phones every minute, to stop mindlessly scrolling Instagram to compare ourselves to others, and most importantly, to live in the now. It might sound clichéd, but it took something so unimaginably devastating and horrific for me to realize what that means. I wake up crying, and I cry throughout the entire day until it's time for bed. This has been so hard for me. As someone who lives with anxiety and depression, I'm the lowest I have ever been. To be honest, I didn't even know there was a low as low as this.

My husband is incredible, and we are both trying our very best to get through this together. He has a much better outlook than I do, but everyone grieves differently. He said something so wise to me the other day: "How can I sit at home and not live my life when the whole reason we feel this sadness is because Sloane wasn't able to live? We have to live for Sloane. Her life was taken away from her, but ours wasn't." All day long, I juggle between being sad, mad, and angry; I self-blame and ask why me?—it never stops in my head. I know that it will get easier with time. She will always be in my heart, and I will never forget her. I'll learn to cope and live life. But right now, it's impossible to see that light at the end of the tunnel. Sometimes I wish it had been me instead of her, which seems so unfair to say, especially to my amazing husband whom I love so damn much. But this pain of losing a child who I carried for nine months, who took her last breath in my arms, is unbearable. I only got to see her for ten minutes. Ten full minutes after waiting nine months to see and hold my beautiful daughter. I will hopefully have more babies, but they won't be Sloane. Even though I have so many people around me who are supporting me, I feel so alone. It's impossible to feel anything else. Everyone around me is either pregnant or having babies. My hope is that someone who has gone through this type of loss will find comfort in knowing their feelings are real and that they are not alone.

-Anonymous

From a very young age, it was clear that I was obsessed with babies and that I had a strong motherly trait. I was always caring for others, and I was known as the token "Mother Goose" by my friends. It felt so right when I found out I was pregnant. I was going to be doing what I felt was my true calling in life—being a mother. Best of all, I was going to be doing it with my best friend. The day I lost my son, who passed away thirty minutes post-delivery, I felt like every inch of me shattered into a million little pieces. I truly believed that I was going to be broken forever and that my life had no meaning anymore. With an incredible amount of support and love from our community, that feeling slowly faded with time, and I was able to believe, even for a second, that maybe I would be able to heal and feel happiness once again. Losing a child was the hardest thing that we have gone through. The most difficult part for me was trying to interact with others. I felt like an alien. No matter how hard people tried to say that right thing, I struggled relating my experience. Sometimes I wanted to just yell at the top of my lungs, "My son died; he was ripped out of my arms!" I wanted to say that he was a real human, with a huge head of hair. He had a button nose, almond-shaped eyes, and the fullest cheeks. He looked exactly like my husband; he was beautiful and looked perfect in every way. This loss was a very testing year for my husband and me. In many ways, we both felt like we were going through an identity crisis and that we were stuck in a place between our old and new selves. We felt every emotion in the book from anger to sadness to shame. ***Days go by where I still sob until I fall to the floor.*** I have flashbacks where I hear myself screaming like a wounded animal in the hospital. While we will never again be able to hold our beautiful baby boy in this lifetime, we have been blessed with a guardian angel. I pray that we will always remember him and honor what he has left behind for us—a strong family unit.

-Anonymous

My first pregnancy was a missed miscarriage. It was discovered at eleven weeks, but the baby had died at seven weeks. So, I was nervous going into my second pregnancy. Once I got past the first trimester, I thought we were in the safety zone and were for sure going to have a baby. Everything was progressing totally normally until the anatomy scan at nineteen weeks. My husband took the day off work so that we could be together. We found out that we were having a boy, and we picked his name on our walk home. We had twenty-four hours of happiness. Then the next day when I got home from work, my husband told me the midwife needed to speak to us. My stomach sank. That didn't seem normal. She told us the ultrasound showed brain swelling. She said, "I can't promise you everything is going to be okay, but I can promise you that I will get you an appointment for genetic screening and a higher-level ultrasound as quickly as I can." I found that very supportive because she wasn't promising things that she couldn't do—she was focusing on the things she could control. That was on a Friday, and she got us an appointment for the following Monday. We spent the weekend furiously googling and worrying and trying to not worry. At the ultrasound, the radiologist confirmed there was significant brain damage. The room was already dark, but it went completely dark when I started screaming. They left us alone in the dark, and we cried as my husband helped me up. We met with a geneticist and a genetic counselor. They thought the baby had a disorder called the L1CAM mutation, which affects 1 in 35,000 babies, and only boys. It is super rare. They didn't know if he would live to full term—he could die at any moment. He could be stillborn if he made it to full term. And then the part they didn't know—and this was the extra hard part—was that if he lived, he could be both gravely mentally and physically delayed. It became clear to me that they were leaving it to us to decide. I just wanted someone to tell me what to do. I could ride out the pregnancy and see what happened or terminate. We didn't have to decide at that moment, but we had to make a decision pretty quickly, because after a certain number of weeks, it would be illegal to do a medical termination. They sent us home with a booklet with lots of stories of people who were on the same path as we were. I read it over and over again. By the time we had left the appointment, we'd already made the decision. They booked us for our labor and delivery the following week. I wanted my midwife to be at the birth. We wanted everything to be as we envisioned it. After our son was born, it was actually super joyful. Both sets of grandparents got to meet him, and we took pictures of everyone holding him. The nurses would periodically come in and check his vitals. He was going to die at some point, but they didn't know when. It was about three hours after he was born when they said his heart wasn't beating anymore. We didn't want to give him back to the nurses. We just wanted to hold him, but we gave him back at some point and by then he was cold. The next morning, they brought him back for a nonreligious baby-naming ceremony. It was very impactful for us because we wanted some sort of ceremony to mark this baby's entrance and exit from the world. Then we were discharged. We gave him back for good. Before they sent us off, they made us a memorial package with mementos. I had just given birth, so I was wearing granny panties and was bleeding. They also make you wear a sports bra so your milk doesn't come in. ***It was a weird scenario leaving the hospital with nothing but an envelope of pictures of my baby who had died.***

-Anonymous

My mom has end-stage dementia, so when I had my first daughter, I thought I could do everything by myself. I thought that I didn't need anyone. I didn't have my mom, but everyone else had their moms. No one I knew could relate at the time. I was close to my grandmother, but she passed away five years ago. My dad is on another planet, and I'm an only child. I felt like I had no one, and I was in such a bad place because of it. ***I felt extreme isolation and loneliness.*** I wanted to be able to call my mom and say, "This is hard. How did you get through it? What can I do? Can you help me?" I'm not close enough with my mother-in-law to talk about those things. For some reason, having my daughter brought up so much grief. I was not myself for months—it felt like I was in a cloud. I lost a lot of friends who didn't understand. They said, "You should be happy—you have a baby."

-Anonymous

I had a miscarriage during COVID-19, and my experience in the hospital was awful and cold.

I was on my way to my parents' cabin in British Columbia to work remotely. My boyfriend at the time stayed behind in Calgary to work. After about a week at the cabin, I didn't have my period, and I noticed some symptoms that were unusual. I took a test, and I was pregnant. A week later, I went back to Calgary for a doctor's appointment and found out I was about three months pregnant. I did all the tests and saw the little heartbeat. Best moment ever. Later that day, I was not feeling well, and I was bleeding excessively. My mom rushed me to the little hospital in town where I stayed for the night. My mom couldn't even come in with me. After tests and tests, they couldn't find a heartbeat (worst moment of my life). I was transferred to another hospital where I got more tests. I hemorrhaged and had to go under and get extra help. My parents were not informed, and they couldn't help me due to COVID-19. It was the scariest moment of my life. After about thirty hours of being in two hospitals, the doctor informed me I had had a miscarriage. There was no sympathy, empathy, help in any way, or advice provided about what to do next from the doctors or nursing staff. ***I lost my baby that day and no one even cared.*** Then my boyfriend left me the next day. I didn't get out of bed for about three months. I am still having a hard time. I have a tattoo of my baby on my body to remind me of how strong I am. I had a very strong feeling it was a girl—I even named her: Lucky. I thought about her recently, and a double rainbow appeared out of nowhere. I know she is still with me. Even though I never got to meet my baby, I feel like I still had one. I'd never known anyone who had had a miscarriage until it happened to me. It is the single worst thing that can happen to a woman. I felt her heartbeat. I had a life growing in me, and then it was ripped out of me. I still blame myself to this day, and I know I shouldn't, but I find it hard not to. Now I am able to tell my story when it's necessary and to the right person. I feel a lot better when I do. It's part of my healing process.

-Anonymous

I had a miscarriage during quarantine. As if these times were not isolating enough, adding that to the mix is intense. I'm very fortunate to have a son who is almost a year, plus a very supportive husband, but I still feel alone. It's difficult because there is a stigma around telling anyone. If you do, they don't know what to say. But if you don't, you feel like you're hiding something that you're ashamed of. The shame makes it feel like what happened to me is my own fault, which I know it isn't. The first sign that I was miscarrying was spotting. I called my doctor right away. All our appointments were on the phone because of COVID-19, which was weird in itself. My doctor sent me for bloodwork and an ultrasound. It was nerve racking to go to these places during this already scary time. I also had to go to my ultrasound appointment alone because they wouldn't let another person come in. That was a lot. The ultrasound confirmed the miscarriage, which I found out at the clinic. I then had to drive home alone. Because of some possible complications, my doctor referred me to the early pregnancy clinic at the hospital. Again, all my appointments were on the phone. COVID-19 made this experience feel even more lonely because I never saw a doctor face-to-face, and the medical professionals I did see were wearing full gowns, masks, and gloves. I think there might have been more emotional support if I saw someone in person, but my doctor did call and check in on me a few times after the miscarriage, which was comforting. ***There isn't much support or awareness around miscarriage, yet it happens more often than we know.*** It's so confusing because as soon as you find out you're pregnant, you start making plans in your head, and then in the blink of an eye, those plans are derailed. When I first found out I was pregnant, I was worried that we weren't ready for another child, and then when the miscarriage started, I was so anxious and fearful about losing the baby. And now that I've lost the baby, I feel empty and numb. It's a roller coaster of emotions in a short amount of time that can make you feel very lonely. So now I grieve and am giving myself time to heal.

-Anonymous

Becoming a solo parent, after never expecting it, throws everything you think you know into question. Even though I was already on my own with my kids 90 percent of the time, I always had that person I could call, or who I could roll my eyes with at some ridiculous thing the boys were doing—someone who knew their idiosyncrasies as well as I did. It tore me open to my core after that person was gone in a split second. And while it made me question so much of our life and how we could ever feel safe again, it solidified the importance of putting my kids' needs even more in the forefront: ensuring they know, without a doubt, that they are loved unconditionally even though they have one less living parent, and that I will do everything in my power to keep them safe. This was almost impossible when I had trouble feeling safe myself. Feelings are so important while guiding young children through grief—knowing that there is no such thing as good or bad emotions. That we can and will feel them all. And even if they are sometimes uncomfortable, if we allow them to flow through us, they will pass. Grownups get sad and cry, just like kids. We will all feel angry at things we can't control or change. And if we don't let those feelings out, we'll just explode like a balloon with too much air. ***I don't know if it's because I feel a responsibility to raise my boys into men who are in tune and comfortable with their emotions, but I've always felt it's important to normalize all emotions.*** But now, with the deep pain we've had to endure and carry with us, feeling all the things is a survival skill. We constantly speak about how we feel and why. And while we may have to filter some of what we show our kids, I think being real and flawed not only serves them but it also serves us as parents too.

-Anonymous

O ver three years ago, I found out I was pregnant. We were over the moon. I had an ultrasound and all was good, they just wanted to repeat it a few days later because his heart rate was a tad high. The baby had grown every day since, but the repeat ultrasound showed no heartbeat. It didn't make sense. I begged my doctor to do another ultrasound because I was still early in the pregnancy and was feeling horrible symptoms. She reiterated that there was 0 percent chance there was a viable pregnancy. I will never forget the vacant look in her eyes. We discussed my options: a D&C or pill. I made the difficult decision to opt for a D&C, and I thank God I did. I was sent into a room alone without my husband and put to sleep with fentanyl. This particular clinic uses guided ultrasound for the procedure. Not a day goes by that I don't thank his little heart for beating at that second as they had the tools in me ready to scrape him out. I was told that the whole medical team cheered when they heard his heartbeat. They took me off anesthetics, and when I was lucid enough, they told me there was a baby. It had never happened before. It was a long nine months with a lot of angst wondering if there was something wrong and if the anesthetics could have harmed him. Fortunately, he was healthy and perfect. It took me longer than I had originally planned to feel ready for another pregnancy, but I was brave enough to do it again. Two pregnancies and babies later, I'm finally ready to share my story with the world. Please, Mamas: advocate for yourselves. ***As a social worker, I thought I had advocated for myself, but I should have pushed harder for that ultrasound.*** Thank God his tiny heart was detected in the clinic. I know this is rare, but if you're told something that you don't feel in your heart is right, push for more testing. Share this with your friends.

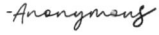

-Anonymous

When my daughter was seven months old, I got pregnant with my son. Two months before that, I found out my mother had lung cancer. She was not a smoker, but obviously this happens. Then I got pregnant. I was not meaning to get pregnant, but it just happened. ***My mother passed away while I was pregnant with my son.*** My husband says that my son saved me. I wouldn't have been able to be a mother to our seven-month-old daughter if I hadn't been pregnant with my son. He was born four months after she died. It was a real thing. She was diagnosed in May, I got pregnant in July, and she died in January. After he was born, I honestly was so exhausted. I was exhausted from the emotional roller coaster of watching my mother die, being that support for her and my family, and having to be strong because I was growing a human being inside me. It was hard for me to find the connection with my son. Every hormone ran out, and I couldn't wrap my head around being a mother without my mother around. I had just become a mother. My daughter was only seventeen months old when my mom died, and she was five months old when my mother found out she was sick. I didn't really even have a moment to process any of it, and so at that point it took me some time. It wasn't until my son turned two, right before I got pregnant with my third, that I started to come into myself and accept myself as being old enough, mature enough, and experienced enough to be a mother. Because now I feel like a mom. Now I am totally a mom. I have a two-year-old son, my daughter is four, and I have three dogs: small, medium, and large. I have an incredible husband (who I want to kill sometimes), but he is the best, and I run a company, so it's okay, right?!

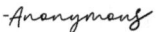

-Anonymous

CLOSING NOTES

Beyond the fourth trimester

you've made it to the end of the book, and you're likely close to the end of your official fourth trimester. Welcome to the other side! As we mentioned in the intro, while the technical definition of postpartum is a short period of time after giving birth, once you've become postpartum, you are never not postpartum. Your body, your mind, and your life has been changed forever. This is why we invite you again to our social channel @this.is.eemah to hear more stories and connect with a village of moms who range from just-had-a-baby to grandparents.

When we started this project in 2018, we knew there was a need for this kind of real conversation about postpartum. We were new moms who came to the table having read all the books and having asked all the questions, and we were still both struck by how many things would surprise us every day. And when you're a new mom in the weeds, the last thing you need is a surprise. You need education, support, and the ability to know how to advocate for your needs and a way to feel connected in a time that is hellbent on making you feel alone.

Because you're not alone, and from two moms of a five-year-old and a seven-year-old, we can safely say, it gets better. From the other side of the postpartum fence, we can tell you that the grass looks greener for a reason. It's hard to feel like you will ever come out of it, but then one day you do. The diapers are gone, your kids can do things on their own (more and more each day), and you get back your time, your capacity, and yourself. We're not saying it doesn't take a lot of work—your new life doesn't just magically happen, but all the things that feel lost can be found again. We spent a collective four years in the weeds of postpartum, and we know how permanent it can seem. We hope that hearing from us, two people who were so traumatized and motivated by postpartum that we devoted four years and a book to it, is reassuring that this too shall pass.

Our hope is that you were able to tell your own story, get it out, and write it down. You are invited (but not obligated) to share any or all of your pages with us at @this.is.eemah where we celebrate the amazing stories of our community. Or you can keep them to yourself to read when you are years out and the memories of this time in your life have blurred. Share them with a friend who has just become a new mom to help her move through her own journey, or never look at them again. Whatever you do with this book, we hope you felt connected, supported, loved, and seen.

We are all truly in this motherhood game together.

XO
Jord and Lani

TELL YOUR STORY . . .

We've left a few pages here in case you have more
to share. Your story matters, so whether you write
it in these pages or share it with a friend, don't shy
away from adding your voice to the conversation
about postpartum.

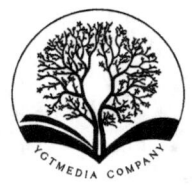

YGTMedia Co. is a blended boutique publishing house for mission-driven humans. We help seasoned and emerging authors "birth their brain babies" through a supportive and collaborative approach. Specializing in narrative nonfiction and adult and children's empowerment books, we believe that words can change the world, and we intend to do so one book at a time.

ygtmedia.co/publishing

@ygtmedia.company

@ygtmedia.co

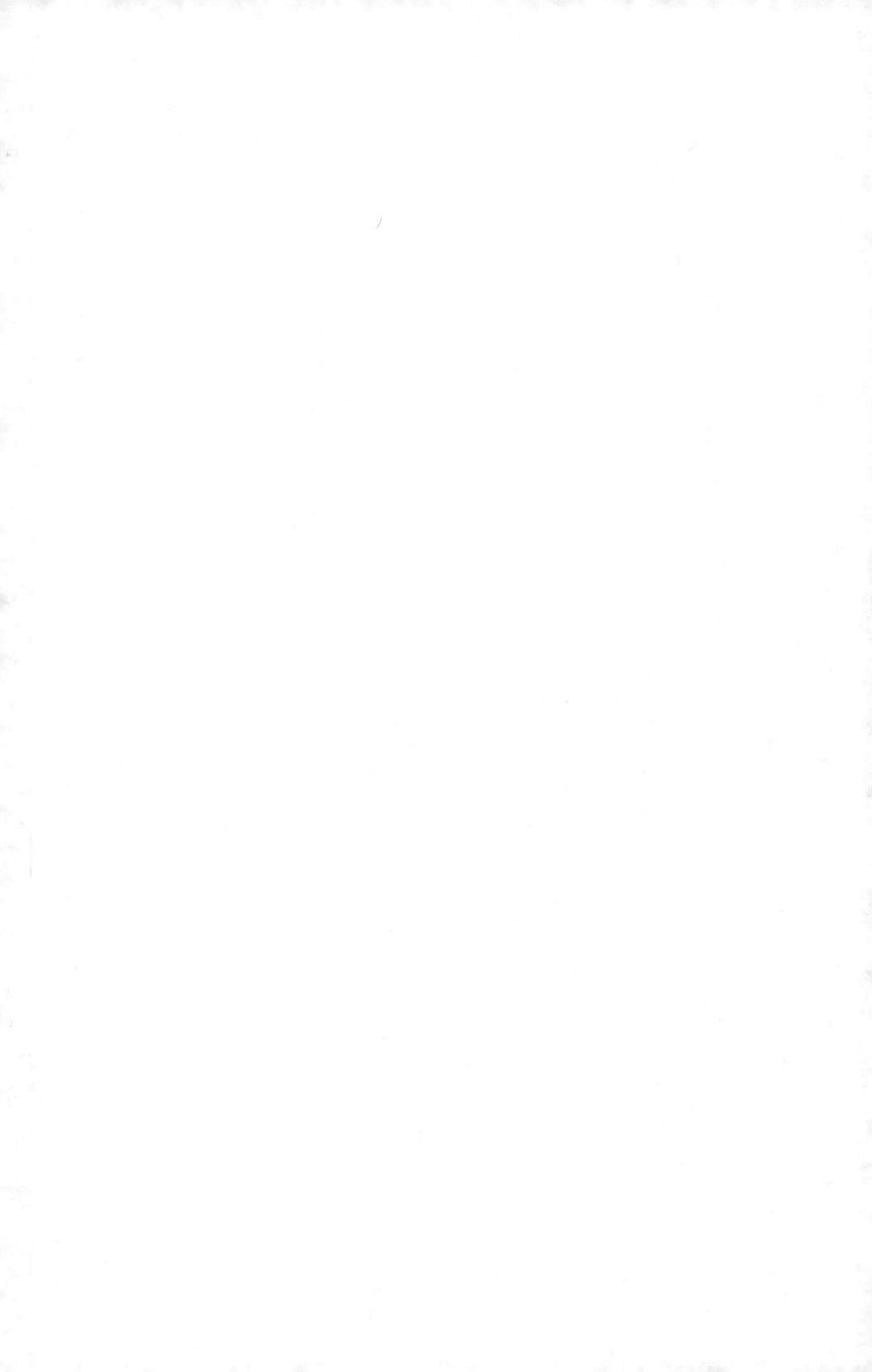

www.ingramcontent.com/pod-product-compliance
Lightning Source LLC
Chambersburg PA
CBHW071144120626
46546CB00006B/2125